# Mental capacity legislation: principles and practice

# Mental capacity legislation: principles and practice

Edited by Rebecca Jacob, Michael Gunn and Anthony Holland

RCPsych Publications

RCPsych Publications is an imprint of the Royal College of Psychiatrists,
17 Belgrave Square, London SW1X 8PG
http://www.rcpsych.ac.uk

British Library Cataloguing-in-Publication Data.
A catalogue record for this book is available from the British Library.
ISBN 978 1 909726 00 0

Distributed in North America by Publishers Storage and Shipping Company.

Printed by Bell & Bain Limited, Glasgow, UK.

# Contents

List of contributors     vii

Foreword by George Szmukler     ix

Preface     xi

1   Introduction     1
    *Rebecca Jacob and Anthony Holland*

2   The assessment of mental capacity     15
    *Matthew Hotopf*

3   Best interests     33
    *Julian C. Hughes*

4   Provisions of the Mental Capacity Act 2005     54
    *Susan F. Welsh*

5   The Deprivation of Liberty Safeguards     78
    *Susan F. Welsh and Amanda Keeling*

6   Clinical ambiguities in the assessment of capacity     96
    *Rebecca Jacob and Elizabeth Fistein*

Index     109

# Contributors

**Dr Elizabeth Fistein** Ethics and Law Curriculum Coordinator, School of Clinical Medicine, University of Cambridge, and Consultant Psychiatrist, Cambridgeshire and Peterborough NHS Foundation Trust, Cambridge, UK

**Professor Michael Gunn** Vice-Chancellor and Chief Executive, Staffordshire University, Beaconside, Stafford, UK

**Professor Anthony Holland** Honorary Consultant Psychiatrist, Cambridgeshire & Peterborough NHS Foundation Trust, and Health Foundation Chair in Learning Disabilities, Cambridge Intellectual and Developmental Disabilities Research Group, University of Cambridge, Cambridge, UK

**Professor Matthew Hotopf** Professor of General Hospital Psychiatry, Department of Psychological Medicine, Institute of Psychiatry, King's College London, UK

**Professor Julian C. Hughes** Consultant in Old Age Psychiatry, Northumbria Healthcare NHS Foundation Trust, and Honorary Professor of Philosophy of Ageing, Institute for Ageing and Health, Newcastle University, Newcastle upon Tyne, UK

**Dr Rebecca Jacob** Consultant Psychiatrist, Fulbourn Hospital, Cambridgeshire & Peterborough NHS Foundation Trust, Cambridge, UK

**Amanda Keeling** PhD Student, School of Law, University of Nottingham, Nottingham, UK

**Dr Susan F. Welsh** Consultant Psychiatrist in Older People's Mental Health, Fulbourn Hospital, Cambridgeshire & Peterborough NHS Foundation Trust, Cambridge, UK

# Foreword

George Szmukler

The contrast between the underlying assumptions of the Mental Capacity Act 2005 (MCA) and the Mental Health Act 1983 (and amended in 2007) (MHA) is stark. The MCA aims to support the patient's autonomy and permits non-consensual treatment only when the person's decision-making capacity is impaired and the intervention is in the person's 'best interests'. Even then, the person must be supported as far as possible to participate in the treatment decision. 'Best interests', although variously defined, emphasise the patient's perspective, asking, for instance, what the patient's decision would have been in their current predicament if their capacity had been retained. Preferences, wishes or values previously expressed by the patient should be explored, including consultation with those who know the patient well and who might be able to cast light on the question. To date, psychiatrists have not been accustomed to this type of thinking.

The MHA, on the other hand, permits involuntary treatment for those with a 'mental disorder' on the basis that the person has such a disorder, and that treatment is warranted in the interests of the person's health or safety, or for the protection of others: nothing about the person's decision-making capability, nor any requirement for the patient's perspective to be given weight in the judgement of their interests.

This conceptual disparity can easily lead to confusion in psychiatric practice. The MCA applies to all patients, those with a 'mental disorder' as well as those with a 'physical disorder', but if the MHA is invoked, its provisions trump those of the MCA. If a person has both a mental disorder and a physical disorder and lacks capacity, different rules pertain to the non-consensual treatment of each. If one type of disorder is a significant cause of the other, whether one of the legal regimes may be considered to cover both conditions may become a conundrum. When the question of a 'deprivation of liberty' arises, the relationship between the provisions of the MHA and the Deprivation of Liberty Safeguards (DoLS) under the MCA seems tortuous.

The clinician badly needs a helping hand in coming to terms with the implications of the MCA for their practice. This is the book that provides it. The Code of Practice accompanying the MCA is a fairly weighty tome, best consulted for guidance (often in conjunction with the now equally weighty MHA Code of Practice) where there is a need to resolve a specific, technical point. The contributors to this book offer a lucid overview of the terrain covered by the MCA, including its sometimes bemusing points of intersection with the MHA, that will serve to orientate the clinician to the Act's underlying philosophy and provide sound guidance to its application. This volume should certainly rank near the top on any list of guides to understanding this new dimension of practice.

*George Szmukler*
*Professor of Psychiatry and Society,*
*Institute of Psychiatry, King's College London, UK*

# Preface

The purpose of this book is to provide psychiatrists and other mental health professionals with guidance when faced with challenging medico-legal dilemmas that require an understanding of both mental capacity and mental health statute. Our intention has been to produce a user-friendly guide to the Mental Capacity Act 2005 (MCA) to be read in conjunction with the MCA Code of Practice.

This book is being published 6 years after the principles of the MCA came into effect and following a period during which mental health professionals have had clinical experience working within this statutory framework. In particular, they have had an opportunity to use the Deprivation of Liberty Safeguards (DoLS) amendment to the MCA in routine clinical practice. Thus, they have been able to draw on clinical experience, case law and the developing research literature regarding its use. The authors include both clinicians and clinical academics, chosen to ensure that practical as well as research considerations pertaining to the statute are taken into account.

The introductory chapter gives an overview of the impetus behind the introduction of mental capacity statute, historical concepts related to its development and a brief description of the provisions of the MCA. The different clinical applications of mental health and mental capacity legislation are also considered. In Chapters 2 and 3, Professors Hotopf and Hughes highlight, in a helpfully practical manner, the clinical application of the functional assessment of capacity and best interests principles. Chapter 4 is a more detailed chapter on the functions of the MCA, which we would suggest readers use as a reference chapter. This is followed, in Chapter 5, by an introduction to DoLS legislation and the burgeoning case law that is arising in the context of its use. Finally, Chapter 6 discusses clinical ambiguities in the application of the MCA, highlighting the difficulties of applying legal statute in a clinical setting.

We thank everyone who has helped us in this endeavour. In particular, Ms Jenny Langdon has provided great practical assistance in the development of the final version. We hope readers find it useful in their clinical practice.

*R. J., M. G. and A. H.*

# CHAPTER 1

# Introduction

Rebecca Jacob and Anthony Holland

In April 2005, the Mental Capacity Act 2005 (MCA), which relates to England and Wales, received Royal Assent, coming into force during 2007. The MCA incorporates into statute law principles and practice that had been established, over many years, through case law. It sets out how mental capacity is defined in law and how 'best interests' should be ascertained when a person lacks the requisite capacity to make the decision in question.

Prior to its introduction, clinicians and carers were in uncertain legal territory when making decisions of a social, medical or financial nature for individuals without capacity. Importantly, however, the Act is more than a solution to a recognised gap in English and Welsh law; it is also about a culture change. It requires those in a caring and/or professional capacity to engage with a person who may lack decision-making capacity, in a manner that involves the person and others important to them in the process of decision-making and has regard to their past and present beliefs and values. The MCA, in its approach, is not so much giving power to others to make decisions, rather it is asking those who have to take a decision on behalf of another to do so in a manner that is transparent, justifiable and respectful of all issues relevant to that person. It is applicable in any situation where someone might lack capacity, from a person transiently incapacitated through excess alcohol or from a head injury requiring treatment, to people with potentially more enduring incapacity due to dementia or intellectual disabilities. It is therefore as relevant in intensive care as it is in social care. The MCA is about the 'here and now', when an immediate decision may have to be made on behalf of a person lacking capacity at the time, but also about planning for the future – how individuals, while they have capacity, can determine who can take decisions on their behalf in the event that they later lose capacity through illness or injury.

Although it was a very significant Act of Parliament, much of what the MCA has brought into practice is what practitioners and others should already have been adhering to on the basis of the developing case law. In its early development work, the Law Commission, a statutory body set up to promote the reform of law in England and Wales, stated that people should be 'enabled and encouraged to take for themselves those decisions they are able to take' (Law Commission, 1991: p. 110). The pivotal concept when determining whether or not the MCA is applicable is therefore whether or not the person having to take the decision has the requisite decision-making capacity. This concept of 'capacity' is defined in the dictionary quite simply as 'the ability or power to do'. In a legal and/or clinical context, this might refer to an individual's ability to make a decision regarding a healthcare matter, undertaking the process of making a will or deciding where to live – in other words, decisions encompassing the social, welfare and health needs of an individual (British Medical Association Ethics Department, 2012).

This book draws on experience gained during the first few years that the MCA has been in force and also considers the Deprivation of Liberty Safeguards (DoLS) amendments to the MCA, which came into force in 2009. It is aimed at psychiatrists and other mental health professionals who treat individuals who lack capacity, and also those called upon to guide and advise colleagues in acute hospitals and residential care settings about the assessment of capacity, DoLS and the appropriate use of best interests principles. In addition, the book considers clinical exemplars in the application of the functional assessment of capacity and highlights medico-legal conundrums faced in the everyday application of the statute.

This first chapter gives an overview of the fundamental ethical and philosophical thinking that has shaped the MCA and a brief description of its historical development and scope. It also compares and contrasts the remit of the Mental Capacity Act 2005 with that of the Mental Health Act 1983 (MHA) as amended in 2007, since there are specific situations when, arguably, either Act might be applicable. Although the Human Rights Act 1998 is not formally dealt with, either in this chapter or in the book as a whole, its principles are clearly interwoven into the fabric of both Acts.

## Medical ethics

A book on the Mental Capacity Act would be incomplete if it made no mention of the guiding principles that have come to underpin medical practice and this statute – sometimes referred to as the 'bioethical' approach. This is concerned with the framework within which a medical decision may be reached on the basis of an individual's views, values and wishes (Harris, 1985), and also how conflicts and dilemmas might be resolved when there are disagreements. Such conflicts may be as extreme as whether or not to start or to continue specific treatments for life-threatening illnesses. However, in essence the clinical situation is described as follows: the doctor advises on the treatment options, taking into account the patient's condition, prognosis and other relevant external factors. The patient, on due consideration, may or may not decide to accept the proposed treatment(s). The moral imperative remains with the doctor, using their medical expertise, to consider all the appropriate steps to seek to diagnose and treat the medical condition and to give the patient sufficient information to make a choice. Even though the competent patient has the absolute right to accept or refuse the treatments offered (except in the case of the assessment and treatment of a mental disorder, where the Mental Health Act might be used to override the refusal of a competent person), barring the most exceptional circumstances, the patient cannot demand a particular treatment (Harris, 1985).

Although a detailed discussion of the philosophical approaches that underlie the development of bioethics is beyond the scope of this book, it is appropriate to consider the theories that have influenced current medical practice. Various ethicists have put forward ideas based on different philosophical principles that have focused on either the rightness or wrongness of the act itself (deontological or Kantian theories), or the extent to which the act promotes good or even bad consequences (utilitarianism). In the former, the essential message is that we should respect an individual's right to autonomy and that each person is treated as an end in themselves, rather than as a means to an end. Deontological theories are concerned less with the consequences or outcome of any act than with the factors that make it morally acceptable, thereby upholding the integrity and beliefs of the individual. In contrast, utilitarianism highlights the moral dilemmas faced when considering the outcome of an act, i.e. the extent to which it leads to positive or negative consequences. This implies that the moral worth of an action is determined only by its resulting outcome. The utilitarian measure of a positive outcome, therefore, is the maximisation of happiness (Mason & Laurie, 2006).

Drawing on these and other philosophical theories, Beauchamp & Childress (2001) have suggested the concept of 'principlism' as a way to resolve medical ethical dilemmas. They broadly argue that the justification for our actions should be based on accepted values. They suggest that ethically appropriate conduct is determined by reference to four key principles, which are to be taken into account when reflecting on one's behaviour towards others. These are:

- the principle of respect for individual autonomy (i.e. individuals must be viewed as independent moral agents with the 'right' to choose how to live their own lives)
- the principle of beneficence (i.e. one should strive to do good where possible)
- the principle of non-maleficence (i.e. one should avoid doing harm to others)
- the principle of justice (i.e. people should be treated fairly, although this does not necessarily equate with treating everyone equally).

The principles of beneficence and non-maleficence are by no means new concepts and their origins extend to the Hippocratic Oath, which states:

'I will prescribe regimens for the good of my patients according to my ability and judgement and never do harm to anyone.'

According to advocates of the four-principles approach, one of its advantages is that, because the principles are independent of any particular philosophical theory, theorists working in a variety of different traditions can use them. However, this approach has been criticised on the basis that it does not offer any clear way of prioritising between the principles in cases where they conflict, as they are liable to do (Savulescu, 2003). The principle of autonomy, for example, might conflict with the principle of beneficence in cases where a competent adult patient refuses to accept life-saving treatment, as will be highlighted in the next section. How then can a medical practitioner respect a patient's right, in this case to allow their life to end, while simultaneously striving to do good, where possible, and at least avoid doing any harm? Current ethical thinking, which is moving away from paternalistic medical practice, indicates that, regardless of the consequences of the treatment, the treatment provider must accept the decision of the recipient. Yet this may not be applicable in all cases, most importantly where a patient does not have the capacity to decide. For this reason, greater clarity is needed regarding the circumstances under which each particular principle takes precedence. Despite these limitations, the principles remain useful as a framework within which to think about moral dilemmas in medicine and the life sciences.

## Autonomy *v.* beneficence

The central notion on which informed choice and the importance of decision-making capacity is based is the principle of autonomy. 'Autonomy' has been variously defined but, in this context, implies self-determination. People are autonomous to the extent that they are able to control their own lives by exercising their own cognitive abilities. The acknowledgement of autonomy has served, in part, to overthrow medical paternalism and has led to the elevation of the patient from being a recipient to being an equal partner in a treatment plan (Kirby, 1983).

In the context of the delivery of healthcare, ethicists consider respect for an individual's autonomy as morally required because it is that individual's life and well-being which are at stake in medical treatment. Respect for human dignity entails that individuals should ultimately determine what their well-being consists of, and therefore what should or should not be done to them in order to achieve it. This conception of autonomy clearly implies that the patient has a 'self' which is capable of determining what should or should not happen – that is, they have a set of values, the sense of what is or is not in their own interests, which may be described as the their 'own' values (Harris, 1985). In prioritising an individual's values, clinicians recognise the importance of the patient's views on illness, dying, death, goals for the future and personal relationships, when making healthcare decisions. These values are highly personal and likely to result from the patient's own experience of life and their own reflections on that experience.

The significance of self-determination and the weight placed on autonomous choice by the courts is clearly evident in case law. As Lord Donaldson stated in the case of *Re T (Adult)* [1992]:

'As I pointed out at the beginning of this judgment, the patient's right of choice exists whether the reasons for making that choice are rational, irrational, unknown or even non-existent. That his choice is contrary to what is to be expected of the vast majority of adults is only relevant if there are other reasons for doubting his capacity to decide.'

Although it is evident that contemporary medical and legal practices broadly embrace the concept of autonomous choice of the individual, it is important to bear in mind that full autonomy and autonomous choices are ideal concepts, which we can, realistically, only attain in partial measure. This is due to factors that may compromise an individual's autonomy, including: difficulties in reasoning, which may be temporary or permanent; the inadequacy and uncertainties of the information available to inform choice; and fluctuations in the stability of an individual's wishes (Harris, 1985). There are also other limitations to the claims of autonomy, such as economic and financial constraints – a fair distribution of resources would clearly not allow unrestricted rights to a single individual. Personal choice must therefore be viewed in the context of the needs of a community as a whole. Notwithstanding these limitations, both the ethical and legal duty lies with the healthcare professional to ensure that these impairments and limitations are minimised when initiating medical interventions.

## Consent and the doctrine of necessity

It is a requirement of English law – specifically the law pertaining to assault and battery – that consent must be obtained before any treatment or procedure involving the patient can be lawfully carried out. This is clearly expressed in a statement by Justice Kirby:

'Nowadays doctors, out of respect for themselves and for their patients, (to say nothing for deference to the law) must increasingly face the obligation of securing informed consent from the patient for the kind of therapeutic treatment proposed' (Kirby, 1983).

Therefore, as a general rule medical treatment, even of a minor nature, should not proceed unless the doctor has first obtained the patient's consent, which may be either expressed or implied. There are nonetheless exceptions to the above rules that are essentially to do with situations such as unconsciousness, where consent cannot be obtained, or disability of the mind or brain, where the person lacks the capacity to make the decision. Until the passing of the MCA, the principle applied to treatment in these cases was that of the necessity doctrine. The basis of this doctrine is that acting out of necessity in the best interests of a patient operates as an alternative defence to that of consent, which remains the preferable defence.

Although the doctrine of necessity arose in relation to emergencies, in many cases this defence could be used when there is not an emergency in the ordinary sense of the word – rather, when the usual defence (i.e. consent) is not available but the treatment is still necessary.

The application of the doctrine of necessity has been clarified by two Canadian cases in which the courts clearly differentiated the overwhelming need for a particular treatment from the mere expediency of such an intervention. In the first case, *Marshall v Curry* [1933], the plaintiff sought damages against a surgeon who had removed a testicle in the course of an operation to repair a hernia. The surgeon stated that the removal was essential to the patient's health and life, as the testicle was diseased. The court held that the removal of the testicle was therefore necessary and could not be done at a later date. In the case of *Murray v McMurchy* [1949], however, the plaintiff succeeded in an action of battery against a doctor who had sterilised her without her consent. In this case, the doctor had discovered, during a Caesarean section, that the condition of the plaintiff's uterus would have made it hazardous for her to go through another pregnancy and he took the decision to tie the fallopian tubes. As there was no pressing medical need for the procedure to be undertaken, the court held that it would have been reasonable to postpone the procedure until the patient's consent could be obtained.

Thus, medical emergencies are not an exception to the process of obtaining consent purely by virtue of their need for either an urgent or an expedient decision to be made. Minimum interventions to preserve life are expected in emergencies, but if there is an expectation that capacity to make a decision may improve, case law, and now statute, require that the healthcare professional consider a delay in treatment if, on medical grounds, it is reasonable and possible to do so. Therefore, prior to the MCA, although consent was legally imperative for all treatment, if that consent was not possible and the intervention was necessary, urgent and/or in the patients' best interests, the doctrine of necessity could justify action in specific clinical situations. When applying this doctrine of necessity, it also had to be demonstrable that treatment could not have waited for the capacity of the individual to recover. It is this concept that is now codified in the MCA. A surgeon working in England and Wales faced now with either of the above dilemmas and a patient who clearly lacks capacity because under a general anaesthetic would have to follow the best interests process, unless urgent and life-saving action is required and the intervention cannot wait. Consequently, it is good practice for surgeons to seek their patients' views as to what they might wish to be done in the event of possible, but unexpected, clinical situations arising while they are under general anaesthetic.

In the UK, current medical and legal thinking incorporates the above approaches to bioethics in resolving ethical dilemmas in the practice of healthcare delivery. This is clearly reflected in emerging legislation, not only in the MCA, which embodies in statute the rights of a competent adult to make decisions for themselves, but also in other legislation, including the Adults with Incapacity (Scotland) Act 2000 and the 2007 amendments to certain aspects of the Mental Health Act 1983, with proposals for more options of community care and less restrictive treatments. These legislative changes go some way in addressing the principles proposed by Beauchamp & Childress (2001) of autonomy, justice, beneficence and non-maleficence.

# Development of mental capacity legislation

Scotland was the first country in the UK to formally enact legislation to enable substitute decision-making under particular circumstances. This is set out in the Adults with Incapacity (Scotland) Act 2000. In England and Wales, development of capacity legislation was driven by a number of factors, including the needs of professionals and carers who required guidance on taking medical, social or financial decisions for people whom they recognised as unable to take such decisions for themselves. One case in particular, *Re F (Mental Patient: Sterilisation)* [1990], stimulated debate about the role of the courts in medical decisions. *Re F* involved the medical sterilisation of a woman lacking mental capacity, who was sexually active and whose family were concerned about an unintended pregnancy. The courts ruling in favour of sterilisation stated that doctors have the power and, in certain circumstances, the duty to treat incapacitous patients provided that the treatment is in their best interests. In this instance, an unplanned pregnancy was not considered to be in F's best interests. Some argued, however, that *Re F* went too far in turning the question of incapacity into a purely medical decision based on the doctrine of necessity. The concern was that 'leaving medical decisions solely to the medical profession might imply that they were to be taken only on medical criteria' (Hoggett, 1994). Hoggett further argued that certain decisions are so important that a court, or at least an independent forum of some sort, should make them.

The reform put forward by the Law Commission in the 1990s focused on the fact that people should be enabled to make decisions for themselves but, under certain conditions, and where it is necessary and in their best interests, someone else should be in a position to make decisions on their behalf. It was recognised that individuals regularly face a wide variety of decisions, in areas ranging from medical and dental treatment, to property and affairs, and broadly how to carry out the activities of everyday life. Most adults can and should make such decisions for themselves, but the Law Commission pointed out that people who are vulnerable and lack capacity should be protected against exploitation in such matters. In a consultation paper titled *Mentally Incapacitated Adults and Decision-Making: An Overview* (Law Commission, 1991), it recommended the introduction of a single, comprehensive piece of legislation to make new provision for people who lack mental capacity. The broad values or aims set out in this consultation paper included the following principles:

- people should be enabled and encouraged to take for themselves decisions that they are able to take
- where it is necessary in their own interests or for the protection of others that someone else should take decisions on their behalf, the intervention should be as limited as possible and concerned to achieve what they themselves would have wanted
- safeguards should be provided against exploitation, neglect and physical, sexual or psychological abuse.

This consultation resulted in the publication of the Green Paper *Who Decides?*, which set out how those without capacity should have the necessary assistance in their decision-making (Lord Chancellor's Department, 1997). The document included recommendations of the Law Commission published in its report on mental incapacity (Law Commission, 1995). The Lord Chancellor's Department received over 4000 responses to this Green Paper, from many sources: charities working for people at risk of lacking capacity; local authorities; doctors; professional organisations; and those working in the law. In light of these responses, the report *Making Decisions* (Lord Chancellor's Department, 1999) set out the Government's proposal to 'reform the law in order to improve and clarify the decision-making process for those who are unable to make decisions for themselves, or who cannot communicate their decisions'. The subsequent Mental Incapacity Bill was examined by a Joint Committee appointed to conduct pre-legislative scrutiny before it went to the floor of both Houses of Parliament for consideration. This Committee, having taken written and oral evidence, made a number of recommendations, including a change from 'Incapacity' to 'Capacity' in the title, a requirement for advocates, and the need for the Act to address the complex issue of research involving people lacking the capacity to consent to participation. The Government accepted many of the recommendations and the Mental Capacity Act received Royal Assent on 7 April 2005, just before the dissolution of Parliament for the general election.

The broad aims of the Law Commission reforms are now embodied in statute. The key principles that underpin the use of the MCA are stated in section 1 of the Act as follows:

'A person must be assumed to have capacity unless it is established that he lacks capacity.

A person is not to be treated as unable to make a decision unless all practicable steps to help him to do so have been taken without success.

A person is not to be treated as unable to make a decision merely because he makes an unwise decision.

An act done, or decision made, under this Act for or on behalf of a person who lacks capacity must be done, or made, in his best interests.

Before the act is done, or the decision made, regard must be had to whether the purpose for which it is needed can be affectively achieved in a way that is less restrictive of the person's rights and freedom of action.'

# Summary of the provisions of the MCA

The provisions of the MCA are discussed in detail in Chapter 4 of this volume, but here we give a brief introduction to some of the significant changes that came about with the Act. The MCA deals broadly with two specific scenarios. The first involves 'acts in connection with care and treatment', in which individuals who lack the capacity to make particular decisions that it would normally be for them to make need those decisions to be made on their behalf. The second concerns the process of competent individuals planning for the future in the event of later incapacity through illness or injury. This involves the following options:

- **Lasting powers of attorney** The MCA allows a person to appoint someone, called an 'attorney' or 'donee', to act on their behalf if they should lose capacity in the future. This is not dissimilar to the previous enduring power of attorney in relation to property and affairs, but the lasting power of attorney also allows people to empower an attorney to make health and welfare decisions.

- **Advance decision-making** In addition to giving professionals and carers legal rights and obligations to ensure that care is provided for those without capacity, the MCA makes provisions for patients to have their own specific wishes respected if they lose capacity. This is addressed by the 'advance decision to refuse treatment'. A person can express their wish as to what should happen if they lose the capacity to make a particular healthcare decision. Advance decisions that state a wish for some particular treatment or other action must be considered, but are not necessarily legally binding. For example, a person cannot insist on something that is impossible when the time comes (e.g. wanting to live with someone who could not or does not wish to care for them), or is medically inappropriate or harmful (e.g. a treatment that is inappropriate for the illness in question). However, valid and applicable advance decisions to *refuse* treatment are legally binding, as they represent an extension of the individual's right to refuse treatment when having capacity.

- Another important development is the introduction of independent mental capacity advocates (IMCAs) for those who have not made a lasting power of attorney. An IMCA can speak on behalf of individuals who are without family or friends to represent their ascertainable wishes. The purpose of the IMCA service is to help vulnerable people who, while lacking capacity, require decisions to be made. Such decisions may range from serious medical treatment to a change of residence – for example, moving to a hospital or care home. National Health Service bodies and local authorities have a duty to consult an IMCA in certain decisions involving people who have no family or friends. An IMCA, unlike a donee under a lasting power of attorney, cannot make a final decision on behalf of a patient; however, they offer independent advice to the professional bodies regarding what they believe is in the patient's best interests.

- During the process of legislative reform, the Law Commission had considered the need for an integrated statutory jurisdiction for making personal, welfare, healthcare and financial decisions on behalf of those lacking capacity and for resolving disputes through a new court system. The importance of this area of jurisdiction was emphasised in the setting up of the Court of Protection, which has jurisdiction relating to the whole MCA. The Court of Protection has the remit of being the final arbiter in matters related to mental capacity, best interests, lasting powers of attorney and other matters in connection with interventions provided for those without capacity to make specific decisions. It deals with decisions concerning property and affairs, as well as health and welfare. It is particularly important in resolving complex or disputed cases involving, for example, whether someone lacks capacity or what is in their best interests. The Court is based in venues in a number of locations across England and Wales and is supported by a central administration in London.

- A new Public Guardian has been created under the MCA. The Public Guardian has several duties and is supported in these by the Office of the Public Guardian. The Office of the Public Guardian is the registering authority for lasting powers of attorney and deputies appointed by the Court of Protection. It also supervises Court of Protection deputies and provides information to help the Court make decisions. The Office of the Public Guardian works together with other agencies, such as the police and Social Services, to respond to any concerns raised about the way in which an attorney or deputy is operating.

## The Mental Health Act and the Mental Capacity Act: overlapping and differentiating criteria

Mental health professionals are perhaps in a unique position in having to observe statute and the Codes of Practice of both the MHA (Department of Health, 2008) and the MCA (Department for Constitutional Affairs, 2007), despite the fact that these two Acts are, debatably, based on different and potentially conflicting principles. The MCA respects the principle of autonomy for capacitous adults and sets out best interests principles regarding the care and treatment of adults who lack capacity to make decisions for themselves. The MHA enables treatment of mental disorder in non-consenting patients, whether or not they have capacity, a fact which has been considered by many to be discriminatory (Department of Health, 1999). The MHA is largely concerned with the circumstances in which a person with a mental disorder can be compulsorily detained for treatment of that disorder. It also sets out the processes that must be followed and the safeguards for patients, to ensure that they are not inappropriately detained in hospital. Using a rather broad description of the purpose of the legislation, it is to ensure that a person with a serious mental disorder can be 'detained in the interests of his own health or safety or with a view to the protection of other persons' (MHA: section 2).

Notwithstanding the many distinctions, there is some commonality in the defining criteria of the two Acts. The MCA defines an individual as lacking capacity 'if at the material time he is unable to make a decision for himself in relation to a matter because of an impairment of, or disturbance in the function of, the mind or brain', and the MHA defines a mental disorder simply as 'any disorder or disability of the mind'. Overlapping principles relate to the requirement to use the least restrictive alternative when considering care and to minimise restrictions on liberty. Both statutes enable clinicians to care for patients who need medical interventions and who either cannot (because of incapacity) or will not, in the case of the MHA, agree to the necessary intervention. The legislation takes into account the wishes of the nearest relative, family or friends, and requires that independent mental capacity advocates and independent mental health advocates are available to speak on behalf of vulnerable individuals if there is no one else to do so, although the final arbiter always remains the treating clinician.

The significant differences therefore relate to the condition for which treatment is required. When health professionals are dealing with the treatment of a mental disorder, mental health legislation (i.e. the MHA) usually, but not always, takes precedence over mental capacity legislation (the MCA and DoLS). When dealing with physical or non-psychiatric treatment of a patient without capacity, mental health legislation, via the MCA, is applicable.

Table 1.1 summarises some of the key legal, and clinical, differences between the two Acts and circumstances under which one or the other might apply (Dimond, 2008).

Occasionally, there is debate as to which of the legal statutes applies, and emerging case law suggests that in several instances, the Court of Protection's opinion is required to provide clarity. *GJ v The Foundation Trust and Others* [2009] is a case in point. Mr GJ, who had diagnoses of vascular dementia, Korsakoff's syndrome due to alcohol misuse, and diabetes, was initially detained in hospital under the MHA for treatment of his mental disorder. In due course, the hospital felt that it would be more appropriate to treat him under mental capacity legislation (as he was primarily receiving nursing care and treatment for his diabetes) and a standard authorisation for DoLS was made. An application was made to the Court of Protection to decide whether he was ineligible to be dealt with via the MCA DoLS on the grounds that his circumstances fell more properly within the scope

**Table 1.1** Main clinical and legal differences between the Mental Capacity Act 2005 and the Mental Health Act 1983 (as amended in 2007)

| | Mental Capacity Act (MCA) | Mental Health Act (MHA) |
|---|---|---|
| Mental capacity | The MCA applies only to those who are unable to make specific decisions | The MHA does not require a lack of capacity |
| Mental disorder | MCA applies only to people with mental disorder who lack the capacity to make the decision in question | The MHA applies only if the patient requires assessment and/or treatment for mental disorder as defined by the Act |
| Best interests | The MCA requires that all decisions be made in the patient's best interests | The MHA does not require decisions to be made in the best interests of the patient and detention may be required for the protection of others |
| Range of treatments | The MCA enables whatever care and treatment is considered to be in the best interests of the patient | The MHA authorises only the administration of treatment for mental disorder, but this has a wide definition and may include feeding and basic care |
| Protections available | The MCA provides protection via the Court of Protection, but an application has to be made to trigger its jurisdiction | The MHA has a wide range of protections, including mental health review tribunals (MHRTs) and managers with responsibilities for making applications to an MHRT if the patient has not done so |
| Restraint | The MCA enables only limited restraint in narrowly defined circumstances (it originally did not permit a loss of liberty within the definition of Article 5 of the Human Rights Act, but this proviso was repealed in the MHA to fill the 'Bournewood gap'[a] and a loss of liberty under the MCA is now possible if the DoLS process has been approved) | The MHA provides the legal framework within which a patient can lose their liberty and be restrained lawfully without any contravention of Article 5 of the Human Rights Act |
| Decision-making if capacity is lost | The MCA recognises several devices for ensuring that decisions are made in accordance with the wishes of a person when they had the requisite mental capacity, to cover situations when capacity is lost; these include advance decisions and lasting powers of attorney | The MHA takes into account advance decisions. Clinical decisions are the responsibility of the responsible clinician; in certain circumstances where a person is unable or unwilling to give consent to treatment for a mental disorder, a second medical opinion must be sought before the treatment can be given |

After Dimond 2008: pp. 295–296. Reproduced with permission of John Wiley & Sons.
a. The Bournewood gap is discussed in Chapter 5.

of the MHA and that he was actively objecting to treatment. The judge resolved the dilemma by clarifying that, if it were not for the treatment of his physical problems, the patient would not be detained; thus, the only reason for detention was for physical treatment. Clearly, this is not within the scope of MHA legislation and the judge held that, although GJ could not be detained under DoLS authorisation purely for the treatment of his mental disorder, he could be so detained in order to receive care and treatment for his physical disorder (diabetes). Consequently, he was eligible to be deprived of his liberty and the MCA rather than MHA was the more appropriate statute in this case.

The judge also highlighted, as a general point, that:

> 'the MHA 1983 has primacy in the sense that the relevant decision makers under both the MHA 1983 and the MCA should approach the questions they have to answer relating to the application of the MHA 1983 on the basis of an assumption that an alternative solution is not available under the MCA'.

It is therefore important that treating clinicians are familiar with the underlying principles of the MCA 2005 and the MHA 1983 and the different clinical situations within which each legislative framework can be applied.

## Conclusion

The MCA is an enabling statute that allows a shift from paternalism towards respect and support of the individual's right to self-determination. However, this shift has highlighted the plight of people who might not consent to treatment, not because they do not want it, but because their mental disability interferes with their decision-making or their ability to communicate a choice. It would clearly be absurd if such people did not receive treatment because they lacked the relevant capacity. Such a situation would open the door to exploitation, neglect and abuse of vulnerable people whose actions and behaviours are compromised owing to unconsciousness, confusion or other reasons, either temporary or permanent. Yet, how can this be resolved without resort to a simplistic approach that equates incapacity to the presence of a particular diagnosis or some other status? And how can those empowered to act in such situations be supported to do so in a way that still respects, as far as possible, individual choice and dignity? It is these issues that the subsequent chapters of this book address in greater detail.

## References

Beauchamp, T. L. & Childress, J. (2001) *Principles of Biomedical Ethics* (5th edn). Oxford University Press.

British Medical Association Ethics Department (2012) *Medical Ethics Today: The BMA's Handbook of Ethics and Law* (3rd edn). BMA.

Department for Constitutional Affairs (2007) *Mental Capacity Act 2005: Code of Practice.* TSO (The Stationery Office).

Department of Health (1999) *Review of the Mental Health Act 1983: Report of the Expert Committee*. Department of Health.

Department of Health (2008) *Code of Practice: Mental Health Act 1983*. TSO (The Stationery Office).

Dimond, B. (2008) *Legal Aspects of Mental Capacity*. Wiley-Blackwell.

Harris, J. (1985) *The Value of Life: An Introduction to Medical Ethics*. Routledge.

Hoggett, B. (1994) Mentally incapacitated adults and decision-making: the Law Commission's Project. In *Decision-Making and Problems of Incompetence* (ed. A. Grubb): pp. 27–40. John Wiley & Sons.

Kirby, M. D. (1983) Informed consent: what does it mean? *Journal of Medical Ethics*, **9**, 69–75.

Law Commission (1991) *Mentally Incapacitated Adults and Decision-Making: An Overview (Consultation Paper No. 119)*. HMSO.

Law Commission (1995) *Mental Incapacity (Law Commission Report No. 231)*. HMSO.

Lord Chancellor's Department (1997) *Who Decides? Making Decisions on Behalf of Mentally Incapacitated Adults*. TSO (The Stationery Office).

Lord Chancellor's Department (1999) *Making Decisions: The Government's Proposals for Making Decisions on Behalf of Mentally Incapacitated Adults*. TSO (The Stationery Office).

Mason, J. K. & Laurie, G. T. (2006 ) *Mason and McCall Smith's Law and Medical Ethics* (7th edn). Oxford University Press.

Savulescu, J. (2003) Festschrift Edition of the *Journal of Medical Ethics* in Honour of Raanan Gillon. *Journal of Medical Ethics*, **29**, 265–266.

## Case law

*GJ v The Foundation Trust and Others* [2009] EWHC 2972 (Fam).

*Marshall v Curry* [1933] 3 DLR 260.

*Murray v McMurchy* [1949] 2 DLR 442.

*Re F (Mental Patient: Sterilisation)* [1990] 2 AC 1.

*Re T (Adult)* [1992] 4 All ER 649.

*Schloendorff v Society of New York Hospital* (1914) 105 NE 92.

# CHAPTER 2

# The assessment of mental capacity

Matthew Hotopf

Psychiatrists are most likely to be called upon to assess mental capacity when a decision relates to treatment or care relating to a patient's general medical condition. This may include medical treatment or the setting in which care is provided. However, psychiatrists are also sometimes asked to assess testamentary capacity: the capacity of a person to run their affairs, or the capacity to form a contract, including marriage. For most of this chapter I will focus on capacity related to treatment decisions. The same principles apply for other decisions.

## When to assess mental capacity

The first principle of the Mental Capacity Act 2005 (MCA) is that capacity should be presumed. However, decision-making difficulties are common both in patients with psychiatric disorders (Bellhouse *et al*, 2003; Cairns *et al*, 2005a; Owen *et al*, 2008) and in general medical settings (Raymont *et al*, 2004). When is it legitimate to question mental capacity and make an assessment? In practice, mental capacity is called into question in three main circumstances:

- when a patient with a known disorder that might impair decision-making (dementia, intellectual disability or severe mental disorder) faces an important decision, where consent is usually explicitly sought
- when a person (with or without known difficulties) makes a decision that seems surprising or unwise
- when a third party (e.g. a relative) raises concerns that the person lacks capacity.

The presumption of capacity places the onus on the agency making the assessment to demonstrate its absence, and the MCA and its Code of Practice (Department for Constitutional Affairs, 2007) are explicit in stating that mental capacity is not to be doubted simply on the basis of an individual's appearance or diagnosis. The point of this principle is clear, and represents the hard-fought battles of groups speaking for people with disabilities to ensure that vulnerable and stigmatised groups have a voice in decision-making. The burden of proof for assessing that someone is lacking capacity is on the 'balance of probabilities'.

The MCA also states (in its third principle) that capacity should not be called into question simply on the basis that a decision appears to be unwise: people are at liberty to make unwise or eccentric decisions. Unless there is a more formal exposition of the mechanisms by which capacity is lacking, the final decision that the individual makes is immaterial. It is not enough to argue that the decision seems unwise or 'crazy', and therefore the individual lacks capacity. However, it seems inevitable that capacity will be called into question if a person is set on making a decision which a clinical team (or other agency) feels is unreasonable.

Who is responsible for making the capacity assessment? Ultimately, the judgement as to whether an individual does not have capacity rests with the agent responsible for implementing the decision. For medical treatment, this means the consultant surgeon or physician responsible for the patient's care. If the decision relates to making a will or entering a contract, it is the solicitor's responsibility to assess capacity. Although the British Medical Association and Law Society guidance (British Medical Association & Law Society, 2009) suggests that all doctors should be able to assess mental capacity, there are circumstances where expert advice and guidance are sought from professionals with specialist knowledge, such as psychiatrists or psychologists. When decisions have major consequences, when there is genuine doubt about capacity or when there is disagreement – for example, between a clinical team and family members – it is legitimate and desirable that mental health professionals are involved in the process, particularly as the available evidence suggests that problems with decision-making are frequently missed by non-specialists (Raymont *et al*, 2004). Ultimately, however, the professional responsible for delivering the treatment is also responsible for making the final decision about the person's capacity.

## Capacity assessments pertain to a specific decision

Capacity assessments can only be made in the context of a specific decision. It would be incorrect to make a blanket statement that a person 'lacks capacity'. Individuals with dementia, intellectual disability and mental disorders may be perfectly capable of making some decisions, but may have impairments to make others. For example, someone with cognitive impairments following a head injury may be able to make decisions on how to spend money for their day-to-day needs, but lack mental capacity to determine how a large payment in compensation for the head injury should be managed. A person with dementia may be able to understand the need to take an antibiotic, but be unable to understand the subtleties of consenting to participate in a randomised controlled trial comparing two treatments for agitation. This is referred to as the 'functional' approach.

The functional approach enshrined in the MCA contrasts with the 'status' approach used in the Mental Health Act 1983 (MHA), and psychiatrists should be familiar with this distinction. Apart from certain exceptions, a patient who has been detained under the MHA can be given any treatment for a mental disorder if the approved clinician thinks it is warranted, irrespective of considerations of mental capacity. This difference in approach is considered by some to be discriminatory (Szmukler & Holloway, 1998): it is as though the presence of a mental disorder of a severity warranting use of the MHA is sufficient to mean that any other decision the patient makes about their mental healthcare is invalid. A further difference between the two laws is that the MCA requires the decision maker to assess best interests and to respect advance directives, whereas no such requirements are made in the MHA.

# How to assess mental capacity

## Information necessary to assess mental capacity

The first step in the process of the assessment is information-gathering. It is necessary to know the nature of the decision to be made, and for this the following pieces of information should be assembled.

### What is the exact nature of the decision that has to be made?

In general hospital settings, it is not uncommon to be asked to assess mental capacity only to find that the clinical team are remarkably vague about the decision to be made. This may reflect hurried communication on a ward round where the harassed junior doctor requesting an assessment has not understood the consultant's request, or it may arise because the clinical situation has changed and what seemed a day before to be a crucial decision has now been reviewed and seems less important. However, it is obvious that the exact nature of the decision has to be clearly defined.

### Has the choice been put to the patient in a straightforward way?

The second principle of the MCA is that all possible steps should be taken to help a person make a decision. There are situations where a clinical team may struggle to give the patient a sufficiently clear understanding of the likely consequences of one or other course of action. Even experienced clinicians may find it difficult to convey the necessary information to a patient when the issues are emotive. Witnessing a member of the clinical team imparting information can be invaluable. It is important to ensure that clinicians do not use euphemisms when describing the consequences of various alternatives. If the patient may die if one course of action is followed, it is important to say so directly.

### Are there a number of options or only two?

Often there is simply a binary decision to be made. In other circumstances a clinical team may be putting the choice to the patient as a simple binary one, but there are more than two feasible alternatives. A surgical team may feel that below-knee amputation is indicated for a patient with diabetic foot disease, because, radical though this treatment is, the chances of wound healing are better. However, there may be alternatives, such as local debridement, and it is important that the risks and benefits of each alternative are understood at the time the assessment is to be made. This is also relevant to determining best interests, as the MCA requires the 'least restrictive' alternative is chosen.

### What risks or benefits are associated with each option and how good is the evidence for these?

Risks are notoriously difficult to communicate to patients, but before assessing capacity it is important to have an understanding of the likely consequences of each course of action. This is not only about risk *per se*, but also about the strength of the evidence relating to a particular risk. For example, the consequences of a patient with diabetic ketoacidosis refusing rehydration and correction of hyperglycaemia is far better understood than those of a patient with advanced cancer not having second-line palliative chemotherapy. To refuse treatment for diabetic ketoacidosis will inevitably lead to death, and this risk is not just extreme, it is also very well understood. If the treatment proposed is little more than experimental (e.g. some forms of palliative chemotherapy), the risks of refusing it are marginal, but also the evidence that it will lead to benefit is far less well quantified.

### How urgently does the decision have to be made?

It is obvious that when a decision has to be made very quickly, there will be less time to gather or present information to the patient. However, there are many situations when urgent capacity assessments are requested, but the decision can be postponed for hours or even days. This not only allows more time for an assessment, but also ensures that, if the person has a fluctuating level of capacity, they can be assessed when they are at their best.

### If the individual is refusing treatment or care, what is the history of this refusal?

Although – strictly speaking – such considerations belong to the assessment of best interests, the approach to assessment will differ depending on the chronicity of the condition and how much time the patient has had to consider the options. Simply because there has been a consistently expressed reluctance to have a procedure in the event of a deteriorating clinical condition (e.g. amputation for diabetic foot disease) should not necessarily mean that mental capacity to refuse is not considered at the time the procedure is indicated. But the refusal is more likely to be a capable one than in a situation where a patient has had very little time to consider the options.

## Is there any barrier to communication, such as deafness or language difficulties, and if so, what steps have been taken to overcome these?

The MCA makes it clear that every reasonable step should be taken to overcome communication barriers. Speech and language therapists or occupational therapists may have special skills to assist patients with communication difficulties. Signing can be used for deaf patients, and interpreters for non-English speakers. Although a patient may have reasonably good English and is usually able to communicate effectively with professionals, if English is not the first language and there is some degree of impairment caused, for example, by mild dementia, communication may be more effective in the patient's mother tongue. Further, even patients with excellent English may not always understand the colloquial or euphemistic language so common in medicine (Box 2.1).

## Is there any concern that a patient is being coerced by someone?

Although this is not strictly part of the assessment of mental capacity, there may be many pressures on patients which influence their expressed wishes and which need to be taken into account. Coercion is difficult to define and difficult to assess under these circumstances. Simply because a patient feels under some pressure might not mean that they are being coerced. Thus, for example, it seems reasonable to be forthright and direct with a patient who has taken a serious overdose and who wishes to leave hospital, placing herself at considerable risk, even though she may interpret this approach as coercive. Family members may try to persuade the patient forcibly and it is not always clear where healthy concern stops and undue pressure starts.

However, there are relatively frequent situations in which a carer or family member seems unduly protective of the patient, insists on always being present in the course of discussions and, rather than appearing to

---

**Box 2.1**  Case vignette: communication problems

A young man from North Africa spoke Arabic as his first language, but also spoke English fluently. He had had a long admission for tuberculosis, during which time communication had never seemed a problem. His nutritional status was poor and he had problems swallowing, so a percutaneous endoscopic gastrostomy (PEG) feeding tube was considered. He refused this. A mental capacity assessment was requested. It transpired that he had misunderstood the doctor's description of the procedure, thinking that 'feeding you through a hole in your tummy' meant having a large mouth-like orifice in his abdominal wall. He readily consented after seeing pictures of a PEG tube, and having the procedure explained through an interpreter.

**Box 2.2**  Case vignette: undue family influence

A 64-year-old man had a long history of type II diabetes. He had never had satis-factory control of the disorder, and had run into multiple complications, including renal impairment and foot disease. He had been admitted with a gangrenous sore on his foot, which failed to respond to two courses of antibiotics. The infection was spreading and he had osteomyelitis. He had appeared passive and deferred to his wife, who angrily rejected any attempt to discuss amputation with the patient. She repeatedly appeared to block such discussions and was vocal in her complaints about the hospital's treatment of her husband, as well as in her refusal that the procedure should go ahead. She further blocked attempts to assess her husband's mental capacity. Contact was made with the patient's daughter from a previous marriage, who had a very different perspective and felt that her stepmother was furious about having to care for him and these feelings were influencing her behaviour in relation to the clinical team.

facilitate the patient's decision-making, seems more to block discussion (Box 2.2). Such situations need considerable tact to be handled well, and it may be that the carer or relative simply needs an opportunity to express their views privately to the clinician.

# The definition of mental capacity

## The diagnostic threshold

The MCA takes a two-stage approach in defining mental capacity. In the first place there is a diagnostic threshold. To be considered lacking in mental capacity the individual must have 'an impairment of, or a disturbance in the functioning of, the mind or brain', i.e. a disorder of mind or brain. This diagnostic threshold was introduced to protect healthy individuals who wish to make what others might consider an eccentric decision from having their capacity questioned. The diagnostic threshold is, however, deliberately broad. Thus, although cognitive impairments and mental disorders would obviously be included, so too could temporary states of mind – intoxication, strong emotions or severe pain – which might affect decision-making. I suggest that if the disorder of mind or brain is in this category, the assessor should take particular care to explore why capacity might be impaired. Typical cases include individuals presenting to hospital emergency departments following self-harm (Jacob *et al*, 2005). Many such patients do not have a defined psychiatric disorder, and harm themselves in response to situational crises – such as breakdowns in relationships. Powerful emotions elicited by such crises can, I suggest, impair capacity, but it is prudent to be particularly careful in documenting the nature of an incapable decision when there is a relatively 'weak' disorder of mind or brain, as opposed to 'strong' causes such as dementia or psychosis.

The principle of equal consideration in the MCA states that lack of capacity should not be assumed on the basis of the person's appearance, condition or behaviour. This is a restatement of the first principle of the Act (i.e. that capacity should be assumed), but goes further in making clear that decision makers should not act on prejudices related to the person's ethnic group, mode of dress, condition (e.g. Down syndrome) or behaviour (such as talking loudly).

## The ability to make a decision

The second stage in the capacity assessment is to determine the patient's capacity to make the decision. According to the MCA, there are four reasons why capacity may be lacking. These are that the individual is unable to:

- understand information relevant to the decision
- retain this information
- weigh this information
- express a choice.

### Understanding

Clearly, as already mentioned, the groundwork has to be done to define the decision the patient faces and to ensure that the information has been properly presented to the patient. In assessing understanding, the best strategy is to ask open questions to assess the patient's current understanding, and to supplement this by providing further information as simply as possible before testing again with open questions. Asking 'Do you understand?' and taking the answer at face value is likely to lead to false reassurance.

Box 2.3 gives an example of the sort of approach I recommend. Here, the patient is making a serious decision which will considerably hasten her death. Although it may well be that the demands of haemodialysis are too great for her, and she may be able to make a competent decision to forgo treatment and end her life, given the knowledge of her cognitive state and the seriousness of the decision, the clinician needs to consider carefully whether she has capacity. The interview was attempting to use her knowledge of her current acute illness (pulmonary oedema) to see whether she was able to link this with the consequences of not having dialysis. Superficially, she has some degree of understanding, but this fluctuates over the course of the brief interview. At one point, she links her kidney disease and the pulmonary oedema; at another, she struggles with this. The interview comes to an end with her refusal to continue to discuss the dilemma she faces. On the basis of this extract of an interview, there is at least some evidence that she lacks the understanding necessary to make the decision. However, there is probably a fair amount of time over which

**Box 2.3**   Assessing understanding

The interviewer here is trying to assess understanding in a 75-year-old patient with end-stage renal failure and mild dementia. The patient has refused further dialysis after an episode of fluid overload, which led to pulmonary oedema.

| | |
|---|---|
| *Interviewer* | Can I ask what you understand is wrong with you right now? |
| *Patient* | I came into hospital because my breathing was bad. |
| *Interviewer* | Can you say more about why it was bad? |
| *Patient* | They said it was my lungs, I think. |
| *Interviewer* | Do you have anything else wrong with you? |
| *Patient* | Yes… I have kidney failure. I have dialysis. |
| *Interviewer* | I understand you want to stop the dialysis? |
| *Patient* | Yes. |
| *Interviewer* | Could you explain why? |
| *Patient* | Well… no, not really. It just seems a pain… |
| *Interviewer* | You came into hospital because you were 'fluid overloaded'. That means that your body couldn't get rid of the water you had been drinking and you ended up with fluid in your lungs. This happened because you had missed the last two dialysis sessions. |
| *Patient* | Yes. That's what they said. |
| *Interviewer* | Can you repeat what I've said back to me? |
| *Patient* | Hm… I came into hospital because my lungs were bad… |
| *Interviewer* | … and? |
| *Patient* | … well. Did it have something to do with the kidney problem? |
| *Interviewer* | That's right. The kidney problem means that your lungs can get full of fluid if you're not having treatment. |
| *Patient* | I see. |
| *Interviewer* | Can we just go over that again? |
| *Patient* | I get fluid in my lungs if I don't have the treatment. |
| *Interviewer* | Yes, that's right. Can you explain what will happen to you if you stop dialysis? |
| *Patient* | Well… I would be able to stay at home, and wouldn't have to keep coming to hospital! |
| *Interviewer* | Yes that's right, but do you think you need dialysis? |
| *Patient* | They say I do, but I'm not so sure. |
| *Interviewer* | Go on… |
| *Patient* | Well, I don't feel bad if I miss a day or two… |
| *Interviewer* | OK, but you did end up with fluid overload this time. |
| *Patient* | Well, it was a lung problem. |
| *Interviewer* | [after repeating information that fluid overload leads to breathing problems] Can you just repeat what I've said. |
| *Patient* | [pause] Er. Well, I had a lung problem. |
| *Interviewer* | OK. I'm sorry to be a pain, but I just want to go over this again. Your kidneys don't work, and the doctors have been using the dialysis machine to help your body get rid of the liquid you'd usually get rid of in your urine. If you don't have some sort of treatment for the kidney failure your lungs fill up with fluid. You will eventually die. |
| *Patient* | … hm… |
| *Interviewer* | Can you explain what I've just said. |
| *Patient* | Not now, dear. I'm tired. |

to make an assessment, and the interviewer should return later to continue the interview.

## Retaining information

The second requirement of the MCA is that the patient retains information relevant to the decision. How long does information have to be retained to make a capable decision? The Act is clear that it is not necessary to retain the information over a prolonged period – in other words, if a patient with mild dementia is able to engage in a conversation about a procedure and can retain the information long enough to reach a decision, it is not necessary that she retains it until the next day. The key point is that the information can be retained sufficiently long for the person to be able to use or weigh it, and this may only be a matter of a few minutes.

## Weighing or using information to make a decision

Assessing how well an individual weighs or uses information to make a decision is the most complex part of a capacity assessment. It is the component that is probably most often affected by psychiatric disorders, where delusions and affective states such as depression or mania may affect decision-making. On occasions, strong emotions without formal psychiatric disorders can also act on weighing or using information. It is difficult to operationalise weighing or using information, and most current debate about the nature of mental capacity focuses on these issues in relation to disorders where reasoning and understanding may – at least superficially – be intact, but weighing and using information may not.

Obvious examples where weighing or using information are impaired are disorders (e.g. mania, frontal lobe injuries and intoxication) in which there may be a disturbance of impulse control. The patient, although able to understand that a course of action (e.g. treatment refusal or forming a contract) may entail certain risks, responds to these risks in a way that seems too casual or impulsive to suggest proper weighing or using of the information. Box 2.4 gives an example. Here, the patient is well able to understand the nature of the contract he is entering, and also that he has a disorder which might impair his decision-making. He appears set on a course of action that would apparently have grave consequences for him, and his consultant psychiatrist assesses him as lacking capacity to make the decision at that time because he is unable to weigh information in the balance.

In depression, the difficulties may relate more to a set of beliefs or cognitive distortions that lead individuals to deny themselves crucial treatment. Box 2.5 describes a familiar scenario. Here, the patient is able to understand the consequences of not having her overdose treated, but it is likely that her depressive cognitions, including her belief that she is a burden and that her continued existence undesirable to her husband (despite his protestations to the contrary), lead her to struggle to use or weigh information.

**23**

---

**Box 2.4**  Case vignette: weighing information in mania

A 38-year-old man with a bipolar illness is admitted compulsorily to a psychiatric unit during a manic episode. He is of above-average intelligence, and is difficult to manage. His mood is elated, he is irritable and argumentative about the need for medication. He does not have delusions, and has some insight about his condition, accepting that he is currently manic. During the course of his admission, he indicates that he has made a deal to sell his flat, which he bought jointly with a friend some 10 years before. The friend has long since moved out and has asked to buy the patient out. The consequence of the sale would leave the patient homeless and there is no evidence that he has taken any advice about the value of the property, or the legal consequences of making himself deliberately homeless.

---

In psychosis, the individual may apparently understand the information provided by the clinician, but this information competes with delusions in such a way that it cannot be given appropriate weight. For example, the person may understand the information a doctor provides about the need for surgery, but a persecutory delusion may lead the patient to question the surgeon's motives, believing – for example – that the surgeon is a co-conspirator in a plot. An early definition of mental capacity from case law (*Re C (Adult: Refusal of Treatment*, 1994) included the criterion that the individual had to be able to believe the information given.

### Expressing a choice

In most situations where an individual is unable to express a choice, there will be impairments of other components of decision-making capacity. Most commonly, this will be in coma, where the patient is unable to participate at all. In acute medicine, an individual may not have had time to adapt to a disease that impairs communication. Often, mastering new technologies designed to enhance communication takes time, and it may be that a patient can process the information to make a choice, but is unable to communicate

---

**Box 2.5**  Case vignette: weighing information in depression

A 72-year-old woman was diagnosed with breast cancer 6 years before. This was apparently successfully treated, but 3 months ago a recurrence was diagnosed. The cancer was thought to be relatively slow growing and her life expectancy could have been up to 2 years. She presented to the emergency department having taken an overdose of paracetamol. She expressed a wish to die. She understood that if the overdose was not treated she would die. She was found to be profoundly depressed, with a strong belief that she was a burden, her life was meaningless and she needed to spare her family from unnecessary suffering.

---

it in the short window of time necessary. In such cases, not being able to express a choice would be grounds to indicate that someone lacked capacity. However, there are extreme situations where there is sound reason to believe a patient can understand, retain, use and weigh information but is incapable of expressing a choice, despite all efforts to assist communication. The most pure form of this is 'locked-in syndrome' – a condition usually caused by a stroke affecting the brain stem and leading to complete muscle paralysis. The individual is aware and awake, but is quadriplegic and unable to communicate.

## What does the research literature tell us about assessing mental capacity?

Laws apply to specific jurisdictions, and the English legal definition of mental capacity differs from definitions of mental capacity used elsewhere. It is worth exploring the differences and similarities between our legal definition and those derived in other settings, before exploring whether the wider research literature is of assistance in the assessment of capacity.

The most influential research on mental capacity comes from the US programme funded by the MacArthur Foundation and led by Paul Appelbaum and Thomas Grisso (Grisso & Appelbaum, 1995, 1998a). This work started with an analysis of US case law, which developed the definition of mental capacity to include four domains: the ability to understand, the ability to appreciate, the ability to reason and the ability to express a choice. The first and fourth of these are identical to the first and fourth criteria of the English legal definition (Table 2.1). There is no equivalent in the Grisso & Appelbaum definition of 'retention' of information, but it would be subsumed under their heading of understanding. Appreciation and reasoning map loosely onto using or weighing information in the English definition.

Appreciation is the ability to put information one has understood into one's personal context, in acknowledging either the nature of the disorder for which treatment is proposed or the consequences of the disorder and its

Table 2.1 Comparison of the domains of mental capacity in English and US definitions

| Mental Capacity Act 1983 definition | MacArthur Foundation definition |
| --- | --- |
| Understanding | Understanding |
| Retention | |
| Using or weighing | Appreciation |
| | Reasoning |
| Expressing a choice | Expressing a choice |

treatment. As such, it is close to the 'using' criterion in the MCA. A person who cannot believe the information given to them, because of delusions or powerful distortions caused by affective states, cannot appreciate it. The sorts of questions suggested by Grisso & Appelbaum to explore appreciation include: 'What is the treatment likely to do for you?', 'Why do you think it will have that effect?' and 'Why do you think your doctor has recommended this treatment for you?' (Grisso & Appelbaum, 1998a).

Reasoning is the ability to manipulate information to arrive at a decision. The focus of the reasoning requirement is the way in which information is processed. Grisso & Appelbaum point out that reasoning does not imply a 'Spock-like' ideal of logic – and indeed others have suggested that Mr Spock of *Star Trek* would, by virtue of his unemotional disposition, have lacked capacity (Charland, 1998). In making an assessment of reasoning, relevant factors are that the patient is: sufficiently problem-focused to stick to the task; able to consider the options; able to consider the consequences of those options; able to consider the likelihood and seriousness of the consequences; and able to deliberate. Reasoning is therefore close to the 'weighing' criterion of the MCA. The sorts of questions that Grisso & Appelbaum suggest to assess reasoning include: 'Tell me how you reached the decision to accept the recommended treatment', 'What were the factors that were important to you in reaching the decision?' and 'How did you balance those factors?'(Grisso & Appelbaum, 1998a).

For the purposes of this discussion, the importance of Grisso & Appelbaum's work is their development of a semi-structured interview, the MacArthur Competence Assessment Tool for Treatment (MacCAT-T), which takes about 15 minutes to administer, and questions the patient on each of the key underlying constructs (Grisso et al, 1997). Box 2.6 gives

---

**Box 2.6** Sample questions from the MacCAT-T

*Understanding*

'Please explain in your own words what I've said about this treatment.'

*Appreciation*

'You might or might not decide that this is the treatment you want – we'll talk about it later. But do you think it's possible that this treatment might be of benefit to you?'

*Reasoning*

'You think that [state patient's choice] might be best. Tell me what makes that seem better than the other options we've discussed.'

(Grisso & Appelbaum, 1998b)

examples of the questions used in the interview (which can be followed by further probing by the interviewer). The MacCAT-T manual (Grisso & Appelbaum, 1998b) gives guidance on how to score the patient on each domain, but the instrument does not provide a single binary ('present' or 'absent') assessment of mental capacity.

Although a wide range of alternative capacity assessments have been developed, they tend mainly to focus on understanding (Roth et al, 1982; Janofsky et al, 1992; Bean et al, 1994; Edelstein, 2000). Many provide vignettes on which the patient is questioned, but these do not allow an assessment of appreciation, because the vignette applies to another person and may well lack salience to the patient.

## Reliability of capacity assessments

A review of mental capacity assessment in psychiatric patients showed that psychiatrists can, in the main, make highly reliable assessments (Okai et al, 2007). For example, Cairns et al (2005b) showed that two psychiatrists reached agreement over 90% of the time when they rated a person's mental capacity using the MacCAT-T as a clinical aid. Taking agreement by chance into account, the interrater reliability remained very high. Others have found similarly good results when using clinical assessment aids (e.g. Roth et al, 1982; Bellhouse et al, 2003; Raymont et al, 2007). However, the picture is less encouraging when doctors do not use clinical aids in making assessments (e.g. Vollmann et al, 2003; Cairns et al, 2005b; Beckett & Chaplin, 2006), indicating how clinical practice can potentially be improved by such methods. Reliable and valid assessments of mental capacity are most likely to come about if the clinician either uses an established interview such as the MacCAT-T, or considers each aspect of the legal definition of mental capacity in turn and is satisfied that the patient has been assessed on each criterion.

## Cognitive tests and mental capacity

There is strong evidence that cognitive impairment is associated with a lack of mental capacity, but the two do not map onto each other perfectly (Marson, 2001). It is possible for a patient with dementia to make a capable decision despite a low score on the Mini-Mental State Examination (MMSE) (Folstein et al, 1975). Tests of cognitive impairment are therefore not a substitute for a proper mental capacity assessment, and to use them as such is against the principle of equal consideration. However, it is entirely reasonable to back up an assessment with the results of such a test. Thus, one might record that the patient has a diagnosis of dementia with a MMSE score of 17, and that this cognitive impairment is evident in her inability to understand and retain information necessary to make a choice. Using the results of a cognitive assessment as an adjunct to the capacity assessment strengthens the clinical assessment.

## *Difficult-to-assess groups*

Debate over the past decade, particularly in relation to the use of a mental capacity criterion in mental health legislation, has raised the problem that mental capacity as defined in the MCA and the MacCAT-T is somehow too 'cognitive' to apply to some difficult groups (e.g. Charland, 2001; Berghmans *et al*, 2004; Breden & Vollmann, 2004). Tan and colleagues have shown how patients with anorexia nervosa are apparently able to understand, appreciate and reason about their disorder, thus satisfying the MacCAT-T criteria for having mental capacity, while at the same time apparently making decisions that many psychiatrists would view as incompetent (Tan *et al*, 2003). The MacCAT-T, in not addressing the effect of values, somehow misses a part of the picture. Describing a single case, Tan argued: 'for Carol the paramount importance of being thin has devalued other aspects of her life, such as relationships, education, and even life itself. This new value system has made her decide that the risk of death is preferable to the prospect of gaining weight' (Tan, 2003). If the consequences of this value system are that the patient chooses to die above gaining weight, does this truly constitute a capacitous decision? It is open to argument whether the patient's ability to use and weigh the information is really intact when such a belief system forces her to choose to die above gaining weight. The central ethical question is whether hers is an autonomous decision. Although the MacCAT-T may not be sufficiently sensitive to make these distinctions, there is an argument to say that this is a problem of measurement, not a problem with the underlying construct of mental capacity. In English case law, judges have been able to make nuanced and subtle rulings in similarly vexed cases (Hotopf, 2006).

There are inevitably some groups of patients for whom the psychopathology is ambiguous and the risks surrounding a treatment decision considerable. A common example is the refusal of treatment following an overdose by individuals with personality disorders or undergoing situational crises (Jacob *et al*, 2005; David *et al*, 2010). Here, the psychopathology may appear insufficient to question someone's mental capacity, and yet the consequences of not acting may lead to the person's death. Although it is of some comfort that most patients who present to emergency departments having attempted suicide do not complete the act in the ensuing year, to assume that someone's desire to die is an indication that they lack capacity contradicts the third principle of the MCA – that a person can make an unwise decision. In most such situations, though, I suggest that a defensible argument can be made that the individual lacks capacity on the basis that strong emotions are interfering with decision-making.

## Thresholds for capacity

Although the underlying psychological processes involved in capacity fall on a spectrum, the ultimate legal and clinical decision to be made is a binary one: 'Does this patient have the capacity to make this decision or not?' Is the threshold for making this judgement the same in all situations, or is it reasonable to make adjustments depending on the nature of the decision? Buchanan & Brock (1990) suggested that the standard of capacity testing should be adjusted according to the gravity of the decision being made. According to their account, a patient who refuses life-saving treatment should have to pass a harder test of their capacity than that required had they accepted it. This is a risk-relative sliding-scale concept of capacity testing which aims to protect patients from harm. It views capacity as functionally tied to risk and it allows there to be a distinction between capacity to consent to treatment and capacity to refuse treatment.

Others (Wicclair, 1991; Cale, 1999; Demarco, 2002) have argued that justifying the risk relativity of capacity assessments on the grounds of protecting patients from harm is paternalistic and ethically unsatisfactory. Instead of tying capacity to risk, these authors tie risky decisions to high cognitive demand and argue that it is for this reason that a more stringent level of capacity be expected for patients who want to do something risky – risky decisions are just cognitively harder decisions. The authors argue that this formulation respects patient autonomy and that capacity is kept conceptually distinct from risk. The difficulty with this account is whether decisions concerning life or death (decisions usually regarded as risky) are necessarily cognitively harder ones in the sense that they require a greater ability to manipulate information than decisions that are considered mundane (Buller, 2001). We can readily acknowledge that they are more profound but they may, in practical terms, be simpler decisions to make.

Another way of formulating risk relativity is to highlight that capacity determination, like any test, carries with it an error margin. According to this view, if a patient decides on something risky, then this error margin starts to become significant in a new way (Demarco, 2002). This is because in a risky situation, to judge mistakenly that a patient lacks capacity results in treatment in the patient's best interests, whereas to judge mistakenly that a patient has capacity may result in serious harm or death which was preventable and which the patient (because they lacked capacity) did not freely will. Thus, the argument runs that the consequences of missing incapacity in a patient making a risky decision are particularly severe. Because of this, it is reasonable to expect that those assessing capacity are surer about capacity when a risky decision has to be made. In practice, this involves seeking more information of relevance to a capacity assessment and this may take more time (Buchanan, 2004).

## Enhancing capacity

The MCA places considerable emphasis on the importance of supporting people in making decisions. The ability of a patient to make a decision represents the match between their capacities (to understand, retain, use, weigh and communicate) and the demands of the task at hand. Some decisions would place considerable demands on most people and many would lack mental capacity; others place relatively slight demands on the person. It is desirable to do everything possible to improve the person's ability to make decisions and this can be done either by reducing the demand of the task or improving their capacities.

First though, it is important to stand back from the situation and not approach it as a capacity assessment. There are naturally some circumstances in which a decision has to be made promptly, but in many others there is ample time, and approaching the patient simply to assess mental capacity may push the clinician and patient into opposing corners. In my experience, it is common for capacity assessments to be requested because a patient has refused treatment, and it is common for patients to refuse treatment because they are fed up with the clinicians looking after them and they are making a legitimate if self-defeating protest. If that is the person's motive, approaching the interview in a legalistic manner is likely to backfire. Instead, the person may need sufficient time to make a protest heard.

Capacity may fluctuate. Some causes of incapacity (such as delirium) may improve over time, and it is good practice to delay a decision until the person has had a chance to be reassessed when the clinical state is better. Similarly, capacity may be affected because the patient has just received bad news about their clinical state and needs a period of adjustment to recover equanimity. Forcing a decision that does not need to be made will reduce the individual's ability to make it.

There may be room for treating the underlying disorder of mind or brain that is interfering with the person's ability to make decisions. An anxious person confronted with a major decision may be unable to think it through, but may be helped by an anxiolytic. Similarly, severe pain may affect decision-making capacity, and treating it can help improve the person's capacity.

Information should be given to the person in as understandable a manner as possible. Written information that can be digested outside of an anxiety-provoking consultation may help. Diagrams, photographs and videos can all help the person better understand what is being proposed. Similarly, interpreters should be used if the person has difficulties understanding English.

A range of environmental measures can enhance decision-making. The conversation is best conducted in a quiet, private room where the person will be able to ask embarrassing questions without fear of being overheard. It may well be appropriate to include family members, friends or carers whom the patient trusts.

There is now evidence that such strategies can improve mental capacity (Wong *et al*, 2000; Jacob *et al*, 2005). A well-conducted capacity assessment can therefore become a therapeutic intervention.

# References

Bean, G., Nishisato, S., Rector, N. A., *et al* (1994) The psychometric properties of the Competency Interview Schedule. *Canadian Journal of Psychiatry*, **39**, 368–376.

Beckett, J. & Chaplin, R. (2006) Capacity to consent to treatment in patients with acute mania. *Psychiatric Bulletin*, **30**, 419–422.

Bellhouse, J., Holland, A. J., Clare, I. C. H., *et al* (2003) Capacity-based mental health legislation and its impact on clinical practice: 1) admission to hospital. *Journal of Mental Health Law*, **9**, 9–23.

Berghmans, R., Dickenson, D. & Meulen, R. T. (2004) Mental capacity: in search of alternative perspectives. *Health Care Analysis*, **12**, 251–263.

Breden, T. M. & Vollmann, J. (2004) The cognitive based approach of capacity assessment in psychiatry: a philosophical critique of the MacCAT-T. *Health Care Analysis*, **12**, 273–283.

British Medical Association & Law Society (2009) *Assessment of Mental Capacity: A Practical Guide for Doctors and Lawyers* (3rd edn). BMA.

Buchanan, A. (2004) Mental capacity, legal competence and consent to treatment. *Journal of the Royal Society of Medicine*, **97**, 415–420.

Buchanan, A. E. & Brock, D. W. (1990) *Deciding for Others: The Ethics of Surrogate Decision Making*. Cambridge University Press.

Buller, T. (2001) Competence and risk-relativity. *Bioethics*, **15**, 93–109.

Cairns, R., Maddock, C., Buchanan, A., *et al* (2005a) Prevalence and predictors of mental incapacity in psychiatric in-patients. *British Journal of Psychiatry*, **187**, 379–385.

Cairns, R., Maddock, C., Buchanan, A., *et al* (2005b) Reliability of mental capacity assessments in psychiatric in-patients. *British Journal of Psychiatry*, **187**, 372–378.

Cale, G. S. (1999) Risk-related standards of competence. *Bioethics*, **13**, 131–153.

Charland, L. C. (1998) Is Mr. Spock mentally competent? Competence to consent and emotion. *Philosophy, Psychiatry and Psychology*, **5**, 67–81.

Charland, L. C. (2001) Mental competence and value: the problem of normativity in the assessment of decision-making capacity. *Psychiatry, Psychology and Law*, **8**, 135–145.

David, A. S., Hotopf, M., Moran, P., *et al* (2010) Mentally disordered or lacking capacity? Lessons for management of serious deliberate self harm. *BMJ*, **341**, c4489.

Demarco, J. P. (2002) Competence and paternalism. *Bioethics*, **16**, 231–245.

Department for Constitutional Affairs (2007) *Mental Capacity Act 2005: Code of Practice*. TSO (The Stationery Office).

Edelstein, B. (2000) Challenges in the assessment of decision making capacity. *Journal of Aging Studies*, **14**, 423–437.

Folstein, M. F., Folstein, S. E. & McHugh, P. R. (1975) 'Mini-mental state': a practical method for grading the cognitive state of patients for the clinician. *Journal of Psychiatric Research*, **12**, 189–198.

Grisso, T. & Appelbaum, P. S. (1995) MacArthur Treatment Competence Study. *Journal of the American Psychiatric Nurses Association*, **1**, 125–127.

Grisso, T. & Appelbaum, P. S. (1998a) *Assessing Competence to Consent to Treatment: A Guide for Physicians and Other Health Professionals*. Oxford University Press.

Grisso, T. & Appelbaum, P. S. (1998b) *MacArthur Competence Assessment Tool for Treatment (Manual) (MacCAT-T)*. Professional Resource Press.

Grisso, T., Applebaum, P. S. & Hill-Fotouhi, C. (1997) The MacCAT-T: a clinical tool to assess patients' capacities to make treatment decisions. *Psychiatric Services*, **48**, 1415–1419.

Hotopf, M. (2006) Mental capacity and empirical research. *Journal of Mental Health*, **15**, 1–16.

Jacob, R., Clare, I. C. H., Holland, A. J., *et al* (2005) Self-harm, capacity, and refusal of treatment: implications for emergency medical practice. A prospective observational study. *Emergency Medicine Journal*, **22**, 799–802.

Janofsky, J. S., McCarthy, R. J. & Folstein, M. F. (1992) The Hopkins Competency Assessment Test: a brief method for evaluating patients' capacity to give informed consent. *Hospital & Community Psychiatry*, **43**, 132–136.

Marson, D. C. (2001) Loss of competency in Alzheimer's disease: conceptual and psychometric approaches. *International Journal of Law and Psychiatry*, **24**, 267–283.

Okai, D., Owen, G., McGuire, H., *et al* (2007) Mental capacity in psychiatric patients: a systematic review. *British Journal of Psychiatry*, **191**, 291–297.

Owen, G. S., Richardson, G., David, A. S., *et al* (2008) Mental capacity to make decisions on treatment in people admitted to psychiatric hospitals: cross sectional study. *BMJ*, **337**, a448.

Raymont, V., Bingley, W., Buchanan, A., *et al* (2004) Prevalence of mental incapacity in medical in-patients and associated risk factors: cross-sectional study. *Lancet*, **364**, 1421–1427.

Raymont, V., Buchanan, A., David, A. S., *et al* (2007) The inter-rater reliability of mental capacity assessments. *International Journal of Law and Psychiatry*, **30**, 112–117.

Roth, L. H., Lidz, C. W., Meisel, A., *et al* (1982) Competency to decide about treatment or research. *International Journal of Law and Psychiatry*, **5**, 29–50.

Szmukler, G. & Holloway, F. (1998) Mental health legislation is now a harmful anachronism. *Psychiatric Bulletin*, **22**, 662–665.

Tan, J. (2003) The anorexia talking? *Lancet*, **362**, 1246.

Tan, J., Hope, T. & Stewart, A. (2003) Competence to refuse treatment in anorexia nervosa. *International Journal of Law and Psychiatry*, **26**, 697–707.

Vollmann, J., Bauer, A., Danker-Hopfe, H., *et al* (2003) Competence of mentally ill patients: a comparative empirical study. *Psychological Medicine*, **33**, 1463–1471.

Wicclair, M. R. (1991) Patient decision-making capacity and risk. *Bioethics*, **5**, 91–104.

Wong, J. G., Clare, I. C. H., Holland, A. J., *et al* (2000) The capacity of people with a 'mental disability' to make a health care decision. *Psychological Medicine*, **30**, 295–306.

## Case law

*Re C (Adult: Refusal of Treatment)* [1994] 1 All ER 819.

# CHAPTER 3

# Best interests

Julian C. Hughes

At the heart of the Mental Capacity Act 2005 (MCA) lies 'best interests'. As we have seen, one of the key principles of the Act is that, if someone lacks capacity, any decision made on their behalf must be in their best interests:

> 'An act done, or decision made, under this Act for or on behalf of a person who lacks capacity must be done, or made, in his best interests' (section 1, principle 5).

Section 4 of the MCA concerns best interests and sets out certain steps that must be followed in order to determine a person's best interests. Before considering these steps, however, it is worth pausing to reflect on just what the notion of 'best interests' might mean. This should help us to understand the approach taken in the Act.

## What are 'best interests'?

Whereas the MCA defines what it means by a 'lack of capacity', it does not define 'best interests'. The Code of Practice (Department for Constitutional Affairs, 2007) gives some reasons why this is so. 'Best interests' is not defined in the Act:

> 'because so many different types of decisions and actions are covered by the Act, and so many different people and circumstances are affected by it' (para. 5.5).

The implication is that trying to define 'best interests' would be a hopeless task. Clearly, the notion implies whatever is best for the person. But it is not immediately apparent how this should be determined. For one thing, it might depend on the perspective from which 'what is best' is judged. We can easily imagine a scenario in which what the person thinks is best might differ from what the person's family thinks is best (say, for instance, the person has cancer and has been offered chemotherapy that will not cure the disease but will prolong life by a matter of a few months). We can also imagine a patient and a doctor having different views about what might be best (perhaps, in some other form of cancer, there are good grounds for thinking that radical surgery would be curative, so the doctors are encouraging it). In both these cases we can imagine the family and the doctor putting the case very genuinely that it would be best if the person were to accept the palliative chemotherapy in the one case, or the curative surgery in the other. From a neutral perspective it is simply not possible to say definitively who is right and who is wrong. There may be objective facts supporting the arguments about what is best (e.g. 'the cure rate from this form of surgery is 80%'), but there are also subjective arguments (e.g. 'I just cannot face the prospect of mutilating surgery which will take months to get over'). All sorts of other arguments might come into the equation, but in the end a particular perspective must be taken: a particular individual's view must hold sway. It is not unreasonable to say that the view of the person whom the action or decision concerns should be the one that counts:

> 'People with capacity are able to decide for themselves what they want to do. When they do this, they might choose an option that other people don't think is in their best interests. That is their choice and does not, in itself, mean that they lack capacity to make those decisions' (Department for Constitutional Affairs, 2007: para. 5.3).

Accordingly, the person concerning whom acts are being done or decisions made should be centre stage: their views are what counts, just as they would do if they had capacity. Therefore:

- anyone making a decision for someone who lacks capacity should do so from the perspective of that person
- the key question will always be: what would the person have decided under these circumstances?

This is known as a 'substituted judgement'. In other words, if you are the decision maker for someone who lacks capacity, your duty is to act as their substitute in a very literal sense. Setting aside your own feelings, beliefs and values, you should substitute their wishes and feelings, their beliefs and values, along with all the other factors they would be likely to consider.

This is in contrast to 'proxy decision-making', in which someone else makes the decision, but where the emphasis is not on them taking the view of the person concerned. They might, for instance, take a broader view to reflect the interests of the family. It is important to note that in a substituted judgement this might occur too, but only if it really would be the view that the person would have adopted.

Unsurprisingly, ideas about best interests are contentious. For instance, Hope *et al* (2009) have argued that the MCA is right not to try to define 'best interests', because there are problems with any particular conception of what this might mean. The difficulty stems from the person's lack of capacity, which means that we can never be absolutely sure what they would have wanted under present circumstances. Indeed, even this way of framing the problem is conceptually difficult. For do we refer to the person shortly before they lost capacity? Or do we refer to the person now if (magically) they were to regain capacity? Hope *et al* discuss these possibilities, along with other conceptions of best interests, but conclude that none is really satisfactory.

Given that we set great store on the possibility of autonomous decision-making – in other words we believe that people should, if possible, be at liberty to make their own decisions – substituted judgements seem to be the better option, precisely because they aim to reflect what the person would have chosen had they been able to. The difficulty is that we may have little idea what the person would have wanted under the precise circumstances that apply at the time. (Of course, our certainty increases if the person has made a lasting power of attorney or if they have written an advance refusal of treatment (see Chapter 4, this volume), but even under these circumstances we cannot know for sure.)

Hence, in thinking about best interests we end up with several different strands: there are not only objective facts, but also subjective opinions; there are grounds for thinking that substituted judgements provide the best approach, but they are difficult to work out and know with any certainty; and, meanwhile, it might yet be that a proxy's decision would provide the best way to take things forward in the absence of definite evidence concerning what the person would have wanted. It can reasonably be argued that the MCA, by not defining 'best interests', allows room for all of these factors to be taken into consideration. It does this by providing 'a checklist of common factors that must always be considered by anyone who needs to decide what is in the best interests of a person who lacks capacity in any particular situation'. But the Code of Practice goes on to warn: 'This checklist is only the starting point: in many cases, extra factors will need to be considered' (Department for Constitutional Affairs, 2007: para. 5.6; see also Hope *et al*, 2009).

## The best interests checklist

The MCA sets out steps that should be taken to determine a person's best interests. In the Code of Practice these steps have become known as the best interests checklist (or simply the checklist) and they can be summarised as follows:

- avoid discrimination
- identify all relevant circumstances
- assess whether the person might regain capacity
- encourage participation
- do not be motivated by a desire to bring about the person's death
- find out the person's views
- consult others
- avoid restricting the person's rights
- take all of this into account.

I shall now take each of these steps in turn, to discuss and expand upon them.

> **Box 3.1** Case vignette: Mrs Able and non-discrimination
>
> Mrs Able is a 76-year-old widow admitted to hospital following a large, left-sided cerebral haemorrhage, which has resulted in a dense paralysis affecting her right side. She is currently fluctuating in and out of consciousness, already has evidence of marked speech problems, cannot swallow, dribbles and is incontinent. A decision has to be made about her continuing requirements for artificial nutrition and hydration. Since she lacks capacity to decide for herself, a decision will need to be made in her best interests.
>
> The importance of section 4(1) of the MCA is that, in such circumstances, Mrs Able's age, her stroke and her general dependence are not good enough grounds for deciding on her best interests. It is still incumbent on the medical team looking after her to go through the Code of Practice checklist to determine what might be best for her. If called on for advice, psychiatrists might need to remind those making decisions of this 'principle of equal consideration'.

## Avoiding discrimination

Just as, in section 2 of the MCA, age, appearance, condition or behaviour cannot be taken without further justification to mean that the person lacks capacity, so too, in section 4(1), it is made plain these same factors should not be used to determine what is in someone's best interests. This is sometimes referred to as the 'principle of equal consideration' (Box 3.1). The aim is to avoid discrimination against people who lack capacity, because there is no reason for them to be treated less favourably than anyone else.

The Code of Practice spells out (in para. 5.17) that 'appearance' includes a broad range of physical attributes, 'including skin colour, mode of dress and any visible medical problems, disfiguring scars or other disabilities'. 'Condition' not only refers to physical and intellectual conditions, as well as age-related illnesses, but also to 'temporary conditions (such as drunkenness or unconsciousness)'. Aspects of behaviour include anything that might be unusual to others, such as 'talking too loudly or laughing inappropriately'.

## All relevant circumstances

The Code of Practice very sensibly states:

> 'Because every case – and every decision – is different, the law can't set out all the factors that will need to be taken into account in working out someone's best interests' (Department for Constitutional Affairs, 2007: para. 5.13).

Nevertheless, the MCA itself (in section 4(2)) initially seems quite uncompromising:

'The person making the determination must consider all the relevant circumstances'.

This is made less stringent when 'relevant circumstances' are defined in section 4(11) as those:

'(a) of which the person making the determination is aware, and
(b) which it would be reasonable to regard as relevant.'

The word 'reasonable' appears in a number of places in the MCA. When it does, the effect is certainly not to excuse the individual (in this case, who is determining best interests) from making efforts to find things out, but it does acknowledge that there is a limit to what can reasonably be expected.

Thus, if the best interests decision concerns treatment, it would be reasonable for the doctor to consider the clinical indications, the potential benefits and burdens of the treatment, and the likely outcome of receiving or not receiving it. The more serious the treatment or condition, the more reasonable it would be to consider these issues more broadly. For a major medical condition it might be reasonable to bring in consideration of life expectancy, but this would not be a reasonable matter to consider if the treatment were relatively minor. Similarly, if the decision were a social matter, what might be considered reasonably relevant would depend on the nature of the decision (Box 3.2).

---

**Box 3.2** Case vignette: relevant circumstances and social interventions

Miss Plum is unmarried and lives alone, but now has dementia. Providing a support worker to visit and sometimes take her out would require consideration of her wishes and feelings, as described in the details of the MCA Code of Practice checklist for determining her best interests. It would be relevant that Miss Plum used to enjoy visits to the shops with friends.

If, however, the decision were to do with moving Miss Plum into long-term care, there would be a wider range of issues to consider: the reasons for the move (whether to do with safety or ill health), Miss Plum's attitude to socialising, the geographical location of the home in question, her previous interests and whether the home might be able to accommodate or encourage them, the ease with which her remaining family and friends might be able to visit, and so on.

Geographical location is an example of a factor not overtly mentioned in the checklist, but it is something that it would be 'reasonable to regard as relevant' in making this particular decision and it would, therefore, fall under the description of section 4(2) of the MCA as one of the 'relevant circumstances' that must be considered.

## Regaining capacity

Section 4(3) of the MCA states that the individual determining best interests must consider whether it is likely that the person who lacks capacity might regain it and become able to make the decision in question and, if so, when that might be. The gist of this section is that if a decision can be deferred, it should be. In a real emergency (e.g. to do with medical treatment, or with providing emergency accommodation), by definition, the decision cannot be put off and the duty is to act. But it may be that there is time to spare and, indeed, the person may develop the necessary skills to make the decision with the right support. The Code of Practice lists examples of factors that may indicate the person might regain or develop the appropriate capacity in the future (Department for Constitutional Affairs, 2007: para. 5.28):

- where the cause of the lack of capacity can be treated
- where the lack of capacity is likely to decrease in time (e.g. if caused by medication or alcohol, or sudden shock)
- where there is the possibility of new learning, for instance where a person with intellectual disability acquires new skills or increases understanding by new experiences
- where the person has a condition that causes capacity to come and go (as in some mental illnesses – Box 3.3)
- where the person has been unable to communicate but learns a new way to do so.

## Encourage participation

Just as it states in the third principle of the MCA that 'all practicable steps' must be taken to help people to make decisions for themselves, so

---

**Box 3.3**  Case vignette: Mr Daley and the return of capacity

Mr Daley has a history of bipolar affective disorder and is currently in a manic episode. His speech shows flight of ideas. He is unable to concentrate on any particular subject for more than a few seconds and is constantly on the move. His relapse has been precipitated, as in the past, by his lack of adherence to his medication regimen. But he has accepted hospital admission and is now taking an antipsychotic drug again. There is evidence that his mania is starting to settle. At this point his sister arrives with the news that Mr Daley has just inherited a large sum of money from an aunt. He wishes to invest the money immediately in stocks and shares, but he is assessed as lacking capacity to make such a decision. Instead, it is decided that a decision about what to do with the money in the longer term does not have to be made immediately, but can be put off until he has regained the capacity to make it.

---

**Box 3.4**   Case vignette: joining in with decision-making

Maria, who is 29 years old, has a moderate degree of intellectual disability and has lived for 3 years in a house with two other people with intellectual disabilities. Supportive care is provided throughout the day and night by dedicated staff. Although it is mostly a settled home, every now and again Maria becomes quite agitated and verbally hostile towards her carers and the other two people with whom she lives. These episodes are worrying for all concerned, but they tend to settle fairly quickly.

The lease of the property in which they live is coming to an end and they are being asked to move. It is not thought that Maria or the people with whom she lives have capacity to decide where to live next. An advocate service[a] has been employed to talk with Maria, her family and her co-residents to establish what might be best for them. They start by meeting to discuss where might be a good place to live. They have been encouraged to draw pictures of the type of place they might like to live in. They look at pictures in magazines and newspapers of different houses. They visit different places in the city. They have talked alone to the advocate about the pros and cons of living with other people and about whom they might wish to live with. The advocate helped them to write their thoughts down and they have had a chance to discuss their feelings again at a later meeting. All of the work on the decision has been collated in a big book which they are able to keep and look at when they want. With Maria's permission, the advocate has also talked to Maria's mother to find out her thoughts. By these means, Maria has been encouraged to participate in the decision and the advocate is able to represent her views with her at meetings with her social worker.

a. This is not an example of using an independent mental capacity advocate (IMCA) as laid down in sections 35–41 of the MCA, because in this case Maria does have a mother. Nonetheless, it was felt to be good practice to have an independent voice speaking with and for Maria.

---

too, in connection with best interests, it states that 'so far as reasonably practicable' the individual deciding on best interests must:

> 'permit and encourage the person to participate, or to improve his ability to participate, as fully as possible in any act done for him and any decision affecting him' (MCA: section 4(4)).

It is important to realise that, just because someone lacks capacity, it does not mean they cannot join in decisions that affect them. For instance, a woman with dementia might be judged to lack the capacity to manage her finances, but she might still be able to agree that she needs to go shopping to buy some new clothes and she might enjoy the experience of doing so. Likewise, as shown in Box 3.4, the presence of intellectual disability need not exclude someone from being heard. The MCA encourages this sort of participation.

Using every practicable means to help the person participate might entail fairly simple measures to ensure the person can hear and see whatever is required. There should certainly be attempts to explain matters in terms they will be able to understand. It might be that there is someone close to the person (a friend or relative) who can convey the sort of information that needs to be considered in order to decide what will be best. The Code of Practice (Department for Constitutional Affairs, 2007: para. 5.24) gives the following examples (they are not intended to be exhaustive):

- use simple language and/or illustrations or photographs to help the person understand the options
- ask the person about the decision at a time and place where they are likely to feel relaxed
- break the information down into easy-to-understand points
- use specialist interpreters or signers to aid communication.

## Life-sustaining treatment

At the time the MCA was passed, in April 2005, there was a lot of concern that it would allow or encourage euthanasia – if not active euthanasia, then passively by omission. Section 4(5) of the Act goes some way towards settling these concerns:

> 'Where the determination [of best interests] relates to life-sustaining treatment [the individual making the decision] must not, in considering whether the treatment is in the best interests of the person concerned, be motivated by a desire to bring about his death.'

Towards the end of the MCA, the point is further hammered home. In section 62 it is stated:

> 'For the avoidance of doubt, it is hereby declared that nothing in this Act is to be taken to affect the law relating to murder or manslaughter or the operation of section 2 of the Suicide Act 1961 (c. 60) (assisting suicide).'

This would count against both active euthanasia (where the doctor or carer actively kills the person) and assisted suicide (where the means to bring about the person's death are provided by the doctor or carer, but the person him- or herself takes the final step).

There are two points to consider in the arguments put forward by those worried by the prospect of euthanasia. Both points shed light on aspects of the MCA to do with best interests. First, it is argued that best interests should be characterised more objectively. Instead of talking of wishes and feelings or beliefs and values (see 'The person's views', pp. 44–47), more overt reference should be made to protecting life, preserving health and preventing suffering, which are regarded as more objective aspects of best interests (Society for the Protection of the Unborn Child, 2005). Second, the concern is that the MCA will encourage the pendulum to swing in favour of allowing people to die 'by omission', especially where the person has stipulated that they do not wish to be kept alive, either by way of an advance refusal of treatment or in an advance statement (see p. 45), or via a lasting power of attorney (see Chapter 4, this volume).

These two points are most squarely faced in section 5.31 of the Code of Practice (Department for Constitutional Affairs, 2007), which it is worth quoting at length:

> 'All reasonable steps which are in the person's best interests should be taken to prolong their life. There will be a limited number of cases where treatment is futile, overly burdensome to the patient or where there is no prospect of recovery. In circumstances such as these, it may be that an assessment of best interests leads to the conclusion that it would be in the best interests of the patient to withdraw or withhold life-sustaining treatment, even if this may result in the person's death. The decision-maker must make a decision based on the best interests of the person who lacks capacity.'

The first and last sentences of this passage reaffirm the intention expressed in section 4(5) of the MCA. It has to be understood that when the Act talks of 'best interests' it does not refer to some single aspect that might contribute to a person's best interests; rather, it refers to the outcome of the process of determination. In other words, it refers to everything involved in the best interests checklist. Hence, the decision maker must not consider the person's age and appearance, but must consider 'all the relevant circumstances', and must not be motivated 'by a desire to bring about [the person's] death', and so on. This should go some way towards allaying fears that the Act is not explicitly interested in protecting life, preserving health and preventing suffering. Those who might be tempted to demand active euthanasia are thwarted by the clauses quoted from the Act above specifically prohibiting such action. The Code of Practice is overt about prolonging life, saying that 'all reasonable steps' should be taken, which argues in favour of protecting life. Similarly, if a person is suffering, it is hard not to conceive that this would be one of the 'relevant circumstances' that have to be considered. Furthermore, it seems unlikely that the alleviation of suffering would be something that the person him- or herself (let alone a carer or relative) would oppose. Hence, it is difficult to imagine that the Act would in any sense encourage suffering to be ignored. So there are a number of ways in which it is possible to argue that the MCA is distinctly on the side of protecting life, preserving health and preventing suffering.

However, it might still be a concern that the Act could allow death by intentional omission. As has already been mentioned, a person may stipulate (through a lasting power of attorney, an advance decision to refuse treatment or a statement of values) that they do not wish to be treated under certain circumstances. The real concern is that people should not be left to die when they might otherwise survive. It is easy to imagine how this might occur in the face of very clear prior statements by the person, or by the donee of a lasting power of attorney. And this might amount to euthanasia by omission, as it were, by the back door.

There are four points to note in response, all of which tell us something about the intentions of the MCA. First, as the passage from the Code of Practice quoted above (para. 5.31) makes plain, there will be a 'limited number' of cases where it is right to withdraw or withhold life-sustaining treatment, but this will only be if it is in the person's best interests. As we have seen, best interests has to be interpreted broadly by the application of the best interests checklist, which includes the proviso that the determination of best interests should not 'be motivated by a desire to bring about [the person's] death'. In this sense, the aim of a best interests decision cannot be the death of the person, even if the outcome of the decision is that the person does die. In essence, it can be argued, this makes use of the doctrine of double effect: the intention must always be to pursue the person's best interests, even if a foreseen consequence is that the person will die.

Furthermore, this makes the point, which is often repeated in medical ethics, that there is no real moral difference between doing and not doing something. In this case, whether you are doing something or whether you are withholding something, if you are 'motivated by a desire to bring about [the person's] death', you are breaking the law. The difference between intending something (implied by the idea of being 'motivated by a desire to bring about' something) and foreseeing it is sometimes regarded as mere semantics. But it makes a world of difference. One way to understand this is to consider that whether something is intended or only foreseen is not solely determined by what the individual thinks at the time of doing or not doing whatever it is. The nature of the action itself is also important. A carefully titrated dose of analgesia to relieve pain is quite different from a large intravenous injection of potassium chloride putatively for the same purpose, whatever the doctor may claim they were thinking.

The passage from the Code of Practice makes clear that withdrawing or withholding life-sustaining treatment would be licit only if the treatment were 'futile, overly burdensome to the patient or where there is no prospect of recovery' (para. 5.31). The second point to note, therefore, is that this reflects another long-established doctrine of medical ethics, namely the doctrine of ordinary and extraordinary means. This states that anyone making treatment decisions is bound to take ordinary means to help people, but there is no moral obligation to take extraordinary means. 'Extraordinary' implies a disproportion between an intervention and its likely outcome, for example, a treatment or investigation that is futile or likely to be too burdensome for the patient (Box 3.5). The MCA therefore reflects currently accepted and long-established doctrines of medical ethics concerning when life-sustaining treatments might be denied a person or stopped.

This is not to deny that there are arguments about these doctrines themselves, as might be expected (John, 2007; Takala, 2007; Uniacke, 2007); nor is it to claim that the decisions that have to be made will be straightforward – for further discussion in the context of dementia and older people see Hughes & Baldwin (2006) and Hughes (2007). It is appropriate that there is intellectual debate about principles and doctrines and inevitable that, in a field of complex and conflicting values, working

---

**Box 3.5**   Case vignette: withholding treatment in severe dementia

Mr Jordan has severe dementia and has been totally dependent for all his personal care for a number of years. He is immobile and doubly incontinent and is living in a continuing care unit where he had been placed some years before, when his behaviour was often agitated and occasionally aggressive. He develops symptoms and signs suggestive of a chest infection. Although he has a mild fever, he continues to eat when fed and he is as alert as he has been for some months. His son and daughter have informed the consultant in charge of his care that he was never keen on seeing doctors and did not tend to take medications, even when prescribed, long before he became unwell with dementia. They also know, from things their father said when he was first diagnosed, that he would not wish to be kept alive unnecessarily.

Nevertheless, having reviewed his clinical state and discussed matters with the nurses and with the family, it is felt appropriate to prescribe oral antibiotics on the grounds that they will shorten the course of the chest infection, thereby reducing his suffering. It is not thought that he is likely to die from the infection. Having consulted all concerned and reviewed all of the relevant circumstances, the decision to treat him is made in his best interests.

Five months later, having been a little less responsive for only about a day, Mr Jordan becomes acutely very unwell. He rapidly becomes unresponsive, is diagnosed as having developed pneumonia, probably caused by aspiration, and is soon comatose. Having gone through the best interests checklist, on this occasion it is decided that oral antibiotics are unlikely to be effective, and that intravenous antibiotics (which would necessitate transfer to a medical ward in the nearby hospital) would be burdensome and might still not bring about a recovery. Hence, in his best interests, antibiotic treatment is withheld and palliative measures (tepid sponging and paracetamol) are taken.[a] Mr Jordan dies after 2 days of illness.

a. There is, indeed, evidence that clinicians do make fine distinctions concerning whether antibiotics should be withheld, used palliatively or used with curative intent in cases of pneumonia in dementia (van der Steen *et al*, 2002).

---

out the appropriate action or decision should not be glibly undertaken. Nevertheless, it cannot be said that the MCA ushers in a disregard of basic ethical doctrines or principles. Indeed, to the contrary, it can be argued that the Act ushers in a much needed recognition of the human rights of those who find it difficult to make decisions for themselves for whatever reason.

The third point is that the MCA brings together in statute law much that was scattered in common law. For instance, it should not be forgotten that it has been the case for some while that an advance directive, if valid and applicable, should be followed (see Chapter 4, this volume). Even before the MCA, if a person's views were known, they would have carried some weight and they might have formed the basis for a decision to withdraw or withhold treatment. In turn, this reflects the emphasis given to personal autonomy in medical ethics. If we cherish personal decision-making then, if this is the decision the person would have made, we should honour it (while bearing in mind the caveats that should preclude assisted suicide, manslaughter and murder).

Any verbal or written statements made by the person, therefore, should be given due weight and taken into account (Department for Constitutional Affairs, 2007: paras 5.32, 5.34). But the fourth point is that, in determining best interests, the doctor must always apply the best interests checklist rather than reach an impression on the basis of a single piece of evidence:

> 'Doctors must apply the best interests' checklist and use their professional skills to decide whether life-sustaining treatment is in the person's best interests' (Department for Constitutional Affairs, 2007: para. 5.33).

And it might be that, in making a professional judgement or in applying the checklist, the doctor or other professionals involved feel, perhaps on the basis of an advance refusal, that the decision being taken is not what the person would have wanted and is not, overall, in his or her best interests. Contrariwise, others might feel that the doctor's decision is not in the person's best interests. In either case, the MCA allows that the matter should be settled by the Court of Protection, but only as a last resort (Department for Constitutional Affairs, 2007: 5.33). Indeed, if anyone feels that the person's best interests are not being served, then there is a legal imperative that these doubts should be made plain and considered.

## The person's views

The principles underpinning the MCA make it clear that the person who lacks capacity must be considered centre stage. In determining best interests this is also apparent. 'So far as is reasonably ascertainable', whoever is deciding what might be in a person's best interests must consider:

> '(a) the person's past and present wishes and feelings (and, in particular, any relevant written statement made by him when he had capacity),
> (b) the beliefs and values that would be likely to influence his decision if he had capacity, and
> (c) the other factors that he would be likely to consider if he were able to do so.' (MCA: section 4(6)).

One point to note is the use again of the notion of ascertaining only what might be reasonable (Box 3.6). As the Code of Practice makes clear:

> 'What is available in an emergency will be different to what is available in a non-emergency. But even in an emergency, there may still be an opportunity to try to communicate with the person or his friends or carers' (Department for Constitutional Affairs, 2007: para. 5.39).

The Code of Practice goes on to say that the person's views might be demonstrated by their behaviour; certainly, undue influence should not be used to distort the person's views (para. 5.40). Views can be made known not only by verbal accounts, but also perhaps by audio recordings (para. 5.41), but there is a special emphasis on written records.

---

**Box 3.6** Case vignette: haemorrhagic shock

A young female victim of a car crash is brought into casualty unconscious and with multiple traumas. There is a suspicion that she might be bleeding internally with evidence of increasing shock. She has no form of identification. Decisions to treat her have to be made immediately and it is not possible to delay in order to ascertain what her past wishes and feelings might have been, nor the beliefs and values that might have shaped her decisions about treatment.

---

Written statements need not take a particular form, unless they are advance refusals of life-sustaining treatment (MCA: section 25(5–6)). The importance of the clause in section 4(6) about relevant written statements is that this brings into consideration all advance statements, not just refusals of treatment: hence, the potential importance of what are often called 'values statements'. The Preferred Priorities for Care document highlighted in the Department of Health's (2008) *End of Life Care Strategy* is an example of such a statement. The person can record any values or beliefs that might help someone at a later date to decide what the person would want if they are unable to participate in decision-making. As is well-known, although people can refuse treatment, and under the MCA they can do this in advance, no one has the right to demand specific treatment. However, in a statement of values a person is at liberty to express any views at all, including the view that they might wish treatment to be pursued for as long as possible under all circumstances.

A real example of some relevance here is that of Mr Leslie Burke, who challenged the General Medical Council over its guidance on withdrawing and withholding treatment (General Medical Council, 2002). Mr Burke had spinocerebellar ataxia, a progressive neurodegenerative disorder, and was concerned that he might find himself in a situation in which artificial nutrition and hydration would be withdrawn and he would be unable to communicate his objection to this. Mr Burke lost his case in the Court of Appeal. The Court made it plain that doctors are under no legal obligation to provide treatment at the patient's request if the treatment is not thought to be in the patient's best interests (*R (Burke) v General Medical Council*, 2005). Section 4(6) of the MCA, which stipulates that the person determining best interests 'must consider [...] in particular, any relevant written statement', would have allowed Mr Burke to express his concerns and would have ensured that they were given a good deal of weight. In light of this case, and to take account of the MCA, the GMC has updated its guidance (General Medical Council, 2010).

Nevertheless, any such advance statement would have to be seen in context and it remains the case that the broader notion of best interests implies that those making decisions for someone who lacks capacity should take into account all of the factors that might arise from following the best interests checklist. So, under certain circumstances:

> '[doctors] would not have to follow a written request if they think the specific treatment would be clinically unnecessary or not appropriate for the person's condition, so not in the person's best interests' (Department for Constitutional Affairs, 2007: para. 5.44).

The Code of Practice goes on to note that 'Everybody's values and beliefs influence the decisions they make' and that evidence of someone's beliefs and values might be found in their:

- cultural background
- religious beliefs
- political convictions
- past behaviour or habits.

The vignette in Box 3.7 illustrates this principle.

Section 4(6)(c) of the MCA requires decision makers to consider 'other factors' that the person might have considered if able (Box 3.8). According to the Code of Practice (Department for Constitutional Affairs, 2007):

> 'This might include the effect of the decision on other people, obligations to dependants or the duties of a responsible citizen' (para. 5.47).

So it is permissible to consider actions that might benefit others:

> 'as long as they are in the best interests of the person who lacks capacity to make the decision. [...] "Best interests" goes beyond the person's medical interests' (para. 5.48).

---

**Box 3.7**   Case vignette: Jasmine's depression

Jasmine has a history of recurrent depression. She always attends out-patient appointments with a member of her family and, when she has capacity, she has made it plain that she values family support. The closeness of the family is in keeping with cultural norms for someone of Jasmine's background. On this occasion, she is admitted to hospital with severe depression. She has become almost mute, refusing to talk to anyone. When a multidisciplinary meeting is planned, which Jasmine is invited to attend on the ward, her cousin (who has previously come to out-patients with her) wishes to accompany her. But, although she indicates no objections, Jasmine's consent to her cousin taking part is not forthcoming because she will not communicate. Given that she is unable to communicate a decision, it is deemed that she lacks capacity in this regard and a judgement about best interests has to be made. The team do not feel that anything will be discussed that it might be prejudicial for Jasmine's cousin to hear, they feel it might be supportive for Jasmine herself and, on the basis of their previous knowledge of Jasmine's feelings about being accompanied and of the cultural appropriateness of such support for Jasmine, it is judged in her best interests for her cousin to accompany her during the meeting.

---

---

**Box 3.8** Case vignette: early-onset dementia and genetic testing

A man develops dementia at the age of 46. Four years later, a new genetic marker for some early-onset dementias is discovered, but the man does not have the capacity to give consent for blood to be taken for the purpose of testing him. However, his family are keen to know whether he carries the genetic trait. It might be considered in his best interests to perform the test because it is reasonable to assume that the interests of his dependants would be a factor he would consider if able.

---

The Code of Practice notes (para. 5.48) that courts have previously ruled that wider benefits might include 'providing or gaining emotional support from a close relationship' (Box 3.9).

## Consulting others

The MCA is quite specific about the individuals who must be consulted, 'if it is practicable and appropriate', about what might be in the person's best interests. In particular, individuals should be consulted about the matters mentioned in section 4(6), which concern the person's past and present wishes and feelings, beliefs and values, and other relevant factors (as discussed above). Section 4(7) states:

'The views of the following must be taken into account:
(a)  anyone named by the person as someone to be consulted on the matter in question or on matters of that kind,
(b)  anyone engaged in caring for the person or interested in his welfare,
(c)  any donee of a lasting power of attorney granted by the person, and
(d)  any deputy appointed for the person by the court.'

We are reminded in the Code of Practice that if there is no one to speak about the person's best interests, in some circumstances – where serious

---

**Box 3.9** Case vignette: Down syndrome and the day centre

Jill, a young woman with Down syndrome, has been attending a particular day centre for a couple of years and has built up a friendship with another woman who attends the centre. However, the friend moves house and starts to attend an alternative day centre, which she can be taken to more easily by her relatives. Jill is noticeably dejected. For Jill to attend the alternative day centre to be with her friend she will need to pay extra herself for transport. She lacks the capacity to make decisions about her finances, but it is decided on her behalf that, since she would clearly benefit from the emotional support of being with her friend, it is in her best interests to use her money to get her to the new day centre.

---

medical decisions are being made or decisions that might lead to a change in the person's place of residence – the person may require an independent mental capacity advocate (IMCA) to be appointed (see Chapters 4 and 5, this volume). In paragraphs 5.51 and 5.52, the Code goes on to make a number of points about good practice:

- decision makers must show that they have thought carefully about whom they consult
- decision makers should keep a clear record of their reasons for not speaking to a particular person if they fall within the list given in section 4(7) of the Act
- careful consideration should be given to the views of family carers
- at the end of the process, decision makers should record why they thought the specific decision was in the person's best interests, especially if the decision goes against the views of someone consulted.

The Code of Practice (para. 5.53) suggests two aspects that the decision maker should be enquiring about:

- what the people consulted think is in the person's best interests in the matter in question
- whether those consulted can give information on the person's wishes, feelings, beliefs and values.

The significance of this is that it suggests that the MCA is concerned about both proxy decisions and substituted judgements (see p. 34). The decision maker is to ask what someone 'thinks is in the person's best interests', which is distinct from asking what they think the person would have thought. In other words, although the views of the person who lacks capacity are vitally important, the decision maker needs to be open to the views of others too (Box 3.10).

There are two further points of importance to be noted. First, while it is clear that attorneys appointed under a lasting power of attorney (or an enduring power of attorney), or a deputy appointed by a court must make the decision in connection with the matter they have been appointed to deal with, if practicable and appropriate, they should also be consulted on other issues. They might, for instance, be able to shed light on the person's previous wishes, beliefs, values and feelings. Second, although the thrust of the MCA is that there should be broad consultation to determine the person's best interests, professionals must still abide by codes of practice and guidelines concerning confidentiality. Only appropriate people should be consulted and they should be informed about confidential matters only insofar as is necessary. The best interests of the person without capacity remain central.

At several points already in this chapter, the issue of the views of the family has emerged as important. There is, of course, a relationship between a person's best interests and the best interests of their family. But this relationship is not always straightforward. There might, for instance,

**Box 3.10** Case vignette: agitation and aggression

Mr Hodgson developed dementia 6 years ago. He continues to live with his wife who, like him, is 78 years old. Over the past few months, towards evening, he has become irritable and aggressive. Mr Hodgson's sister-in-law calls every day and is very concerned about her sister. She thinks Mr Hodgson should be in long-term care but Mrs Hodgson is keen to keep her husband at home for as long as possible.

Having had no success with alternative psychosocial strategies, the consultant agrees to try psychotropic medication, having explained the possible side-effects. The response is monitored by the community mental health nurse (CMHN), who has been involved for a long while. Mr Hodgson does indeed show evidence of some side-effects after only a few weeks. Although the irritability and frank aggression have lessened, he is somewhat sedated and slightly unsteady.

In deciding whether or not to continue with the medication, the consultant talks with the CMHN, who feels the situation is less volatile and the side-effects not so severe as to warrant the drug being stopped. The sister-in-law still feels that things are getting too much for her sister and she wants Mr Hodgson to be moved into a care home. When the consultant talks with Mrs Hodgson, she reiterates her desire to keep her husband at home for as long as possible. She is not very concerned about the side-effects and she recalls Mr Hodgson himself saying how he would hate being put in a home. Overall, the consultant also feels that the medication is the best option and, given everyone's views, it is decided that this is in Mr Hodgson's best interests. The reason for not accepting the sister-in-law's view is noted: not only does it not reflect the previous wishes and feelings of Mr Hodgson, nor the current views of Mrs Hodgson, but also keeping him at home, albeit slightly sedated in the evenings, is the least restrictive option and therefore in keeping with one of the principles of the MCA.

be disagreements within a family. Even setting aside the worry that some section of the family might be motivated by malign intent, self-interest may well exist in the most benign atmosphere. If a parent goes into long-term care, for instance, there may be a complex mixture of emotional, financial and social consequences for the family: less to inherit, further to travel for one daughter but less far for another, fewer disturbances at night, resentment expressed by the mother towards her daughter (for not taking her in to live) but not towards her son, and so on. Interests collide and need to be negotiated around the person concerned, who should remain centre stage. In this connection it is interesting to observe that the principles of values-based practice – which emphasise the roles that values play in clinical practice, from diagnosis to treatment – support the importance of thinking broadly about best interests (see Fulford *et al*, 2012).

There is a deeper sense, however, in which the best interests of the person and their family routinely overlap:

> 'interests are often complex and intertwined. In a family, it will rarely be the case that a single person's interests always take priority: rather some

consideration will be given to everyone's interests and some degree of compromise found. The Mental Capacity Act reflects this reality in its broad approach to "best interests". A determination of a person's best interests is not limited simply to what, in the abstract, might seem best for their personal welfare or well-being, but also includes consideration of factors such as their beliefs and values [and] factors they might have taken into account themselves. In many cases this will include strong concern for the welfare of others in their family. [T]here can be no legal or ethical duty to continue caring where this is no longer physically or emotionally viable' (Nuffield Council on Bioethics, 2009: paras 7.35–7.37).

Thus, the Nuffield Council's report recommends that professionals should play a role in supporting family carers to consider their own needs. The philosophical basis for this is the notion of 'relational autonomy'. It is, after all, the notion of 'autonomy' (i.e. self-rule) that places the person centre stage. But, strictly speaking, none of us is entirely autonomous; our autonomy is 'relational'. For we are always situated in a culture, history, geography, social group, legal system and so forth (Hughes, 2001). And we are typically situated in a family, so there is an inevitable sense in which best interests overlap. In a study of family carers of people with dementia, one wife said of her husband, 'My best interests [...] are his best interests' (Hughes *et al*, 2002). Best interests, therefore, do not always collide – they often coincide. Thus, to understand the person's best interests will frequently require an understanding of the family's social and cultural background.

## Restricting rights and acting reasonably

Deciding what is best for a person who lacks capacity can seem like a daunting task. In some ways this is how it should be, and hence it is important that the best interests checklist is followed. However, section 4(9) of the MCA establishes that the decision maker will be acting within the law if he or she 'reasonably believes' that the decision or action 'is in the best interests of the person concerned'.

In fact, the next section (5), entitled 'Acts in connection with care or treatment', sets out that, if 'reasonable steps' have been taken to establish that the person lacks capacity, and if someone giving care or treatment 'reasonably believes' that the person lacks capacity and that the care or treatment is in the person's best interests, then it would be as if the person him- or herself had consented to the treatment. In other words, section 5 of the MCA provides the carer or clinician with protection from liability insofar as the steps taken and the beliefs about the person's capacity and best interests are reasonable.

Continuing the theme of reasonableness, section 6 of the Act allows that a person can be restrained under two circumstances:

- if there is a reasonable belief that it is necessary to restrain the person to prevent them from coming to harm

- if the act of restraint is proportionate to the likelihood of harm and to the seriousness of that harm.

Thus, it might be entirely reasonable to ensure that doors are locked in a home where it would be unsafe for people to go outside unaccompanied. Nevertheless, even if this section allows restraint in the sense of restrictions of liberty, it does not allow deprivation of liberty – a topic discussed in greater detail in Chapter 5 (this volume).

## Making the best interests judgement

Making decisions about a person's best interests might be very straightforward, but it can also be enormously difficult, perhaps because of the complexity of the task (e.g. if there are complicated financial matters to be dealt with), or because of disagreement among those concerned. Given that the number of decisions to be made for someone because of lack of capacity can be vast, there may have to be numerous decision makers. The Code of Practice (Department for Constitutional Affairs, 2007: para. 5.8) suggests various types of decision-making:

- day-to-day decisions by 'the carer most directly involved with the person at the time'
- medical decisions by doctors and other healthcare staff
- nursing decisions or decisions by paid carers
- decisions by attorneys (under a lasting or enduring power of attorney) or deputies appointed by a court.

It also suggests that there will be times when 'a joint decision might be made by a number of people' (para. 5.11). If there are disputes, it will be up to the decision maker to try to reach some form of consensus, not by disregarding anyone's concerns, but by balancing them (para. 6.64). There are various ways in which a decision maker's conclusion might be challenged. Paragraph 5.68 of the Code of Practice sets out the options:

- an advocate might be involved
- a second opinion sought
- a formal or informal 'best interests' case conference could be held
- there could be some form of mediation
- formal complaint procedures might be used
- as a last resort, the matter might be referred to the Court of Protection.

In the main, however, it will be up to the decision maker, who must act in the person's best interests. And the normal way to ensure that this is achieved in a suitably inclusive and broad way is to follow the steps outlined by the best interests checklist. Figure 3.1 depicts the checklist, and what it entails, as a flow diagram. Not every step would be possible or appropriate in every case, but (as we have seen) reasonable steps must be taken before it can reasonably be said that the decision is in a person's best interests.

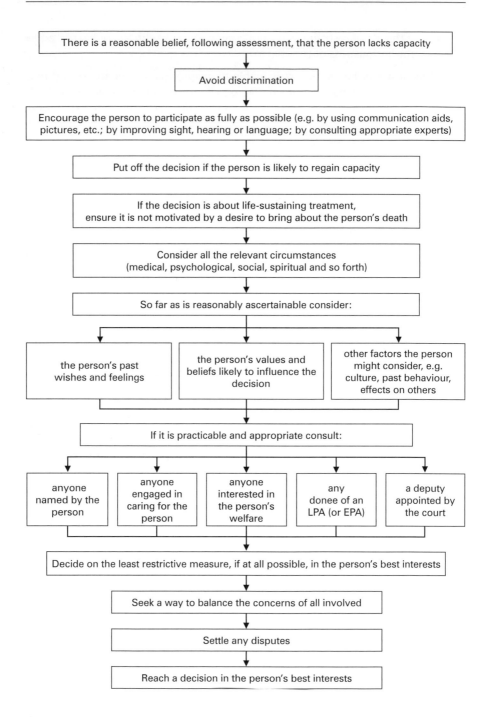

There is a reasonable belief, following assessment, that the person lacks capacity

Avoid discrimination

Encourage the person to participate as fully as possible (e.g. by using communication aids, pictures, etc.; by improving sight, hearing or language; by consulting appropriate experts)

Put off the decision if the person is likely to regain capacity

If the decision is about life-sustaining treatment, ensure it is not motivated by a desire to bring about the person's death

Consider all the relevant circumstances (medical, psychological, social, spiritual and so forth)

So far as is reasonably ascertainable consider:

the person's past wishes and feelings

the person's values and beliefs likely to influence the decision

other factors the person might consider, e.g. culture, past behaviour, effects on others

If it is practicable and appropriate consult:

anyone named by the person

anyone engaged in caring for the person

anyone interested in the person's welfare

any donee of an LPA (or EPA)

a deputy appointed by the court

Decide on the least restrictive measure, if at all possible, in the person's best interests

Seek a way to balance the concerns of all involved

Settle any disputes

Reach a decision in the person's best interests

**Fig. 3.1** Determining best interests. EPA, enduring power of attorney; LPA, lasting power of attorney.

# References

Department for Constitutional Affairs (2007) *Mental Capacity Act 2005: Code of Practice*. TSO (The Stationery Office).

Department of Health (2008) *End of Life Care Strategy: Promoting High Quality Care for All Adults at the End of Life*. Department of Health.

Fulford, K. W. M., Peile, E. & Carroll, H. (2012) *Essential Values-Based Practice: Clinical Stories Linking Science with People*. Cambridge University Press.

General Medical Council (2002) *Withholding and Withdrawing Life-Prolonging Treatments: Good Practice in Decision-Making*. GMC.

General Medical Council (2010) *Treatment and Care towards the End of Life: Good Practice in Decision Making*. GMC.

Hope, T., Slowther, A. & Eccles, J. (2009) Best interests, dementia and the Mental Capacity Act (2005). *Journal of Medical Ethics*, **35**, 733–738.

Hughes, J. C. (2001) Views of the person with dementia. *Journal of Medical Ethics*, **27**, 86–91.

Hughes, J. C. (2007) Ethical issues and health care for older people. In *Principles of Health Care Ethics* (2nd edn) (eds R. Ashcroft, A. Dawson, H. Draper, *et al*), pp. 469–474. John Wiley & Sons.

Hughes, J. C. & Baldwin, C. (2006) *Ethical Issues in Dementia Care: Making Difficult Decisions*. Jessica Kingsley.

Hughes, J. C., Hope, T., Reader, S., *et al* (2002) Dementia and ethics: the views of informal carers. *Journal of the Royal Society of Medicine*, **95**, 242–246.

John, S. D. (2007) Ordinary and extraordinary means. In *Principles of Health Care Ethics* (2nd edn) (eds R. Ashcroft, A. Dawson, H. Draper, *et al*), pp. 269–272. John Wiley & Sons.

Nuffield Council on Bioethics (2009) *Dementia: Ethical Issues*. Nuffield Council on Bioethics.

Society for the Protection of the Unborn Child (2005) *The Mental Capacity Act 2005 Explained*. SPUC.

Takala, T. (2007) Acts and omissions. In *Principles of Health Care Ethics* (2nd edn) (eds R. Ashcroft, A. Dawson, H. Draper, *et al*), pp. 273–276. John Wiley & Sons.

Uniacke, S. (2007) The doctrine of double effect. In *Principles of Health Care Ethics* (2nd edn) (eds R. Ashcroft, A. Dawson, H. Draper, *et al*), pp. 263–268. John Wiley & Sons.

van der Steen, J. T., Ooms, M. E., Mehr, D. R., *et al* (2002) Severe dementia and adverse outcomes of nursing home-acquired pneumonia: evidence for mediation by functional and pathophysiological decline. *Journal of the American Geriatrics Society*, **50**, 439–448.

## *Case law*

R (Burke) v General Medical Council [2005] EWCA Civ 1003.

# CHAPTER 4

# Provisions of the Mental Capacity Act 2005

## Susan F. Welsh

This chapter provides a summary of the Mental Capacity Act 2005 (MCA) and its Code of Practice in certain areas detailed under Part 1 of the Act. More comprehensive details about each aspect of the Act can be found in the relevant sections of the Act and the corresponding summaries in the Code of Practice (Department for Constitutional Affairs, 2007). Referencing is provided where aspects of this chapter stray from the details of the Act and its Code.

Part 1 of the legislative framework of the MCA contains a number of provisions, including those relating to:

- acts in connection with care and treatment – a general (statutory) authority to act reasonably when providing care and treatment (sections 5 and 6)
- provisions for paying for necessities (sections 7 and 8)
- lasting powers of attorney (sections 9–14)
- the jurisdiction of the Court of Protection (sections 15–23)
- advance decisions to refuse treatment (sections 24–26)
- excluded decisions (sections 27–29), including treatment for mental disorder under Part 4 of the Mental Health Act 1983
- research (sections 30–34)
- the independent mental capacity advocate service (sections 35–41)
- codes of practice (section 42)
- codes of practice: procedure (section 43)
- the offence of ill-treatment or neglect (section 44), the ill-treatment or wilful neglect of a person who lacks capacity carries a term of imprisonment of up to 5 years.

Part 2 of the MCA establishes:

- a new superior court of record called the Court of Protection, with its judges and procedures (sections 45–56); this Court provides a definitive legal judgment when necessary, and can determine: the validity or otherwise of any document or decision made regarding a person lacking capacity; an individual's capacity or otherwise to make a particular decision; 'best interests'

- a new statutory official, the Public Guardian, to support the work of the Court (sections 57–60)
- Court of Protection visitors (section 61).

In accordance with sections 42–43 of the MCA, the Code of Practice was issued by the Department of Constitutional Affairs (now the Ministry of Justice) in April 2007, after a period of consultation. It explains the day-to-day operation of the Act and provides useful real-life examples for professionals and non-professionals on how to apply the legislation in practice. The Code has statutory force.

# Introduction

Determination of incapacity has been fully explored in Chapter 2 of this volume. Here I would like to draw attention to a case that recently came before the Court of Protection, *CC v KK and STCC* [2012]. Professionals had judged an elderly woman, KK, as lacking capacity and requiring care in a nursing home, in her 'best interests'. The Judge, Justice Baker, was called upon to determine whether KK did in fact have capacity to make decisions about her care and residence (as well as being asked to determine whether she was, or had been, deprived of her liberty). In his ruling on the case, he confirmed the approach taken by the Court when addressing questions of capacity, which included the following:

- the Court makes the final decision regarding the person's functional ability after considering all of the evidence, and not merely the views of the independent experts (at para. 24);
- professionals and the Court must not be unduly influenced by the 'protection imperative', that is, the perceived need to protect the vulnerable adult, and fail to carry out a detached and objective assessment of capacity (at para. 25);
- the person need only comprehend and weigh the salient details relevant to the decision to be made, not all the peripheral detail; moreover, different people may give different weight to different factors (at para. 22);
- the person must be presented with detailed options so that their capacity to weigh these can be fairly assessed (at para. 68).

# Preliminary provisions

## *Acts in connection with care or treatment*

Sections 5–8 of the MCA cover acts in connection with the care and treatment of people who lack capacity, and provisions for paying for necessities. The following are under a duty to have regard to the Code of Practice when acting or making decisions for a person who lacks capacity:

- people acting in a professional capacity (e.g. a doctor who is assessing a person's capacity to make a particular decision, or a social worker who is arranging for a person to move into supported accommodation)
- people who are being paid for acts or in relation to that person (e.g. a care assistant working in a residential home for people with intellectual disabilities)
- an attorney under a lasting power of attorney
- a deputy appointed by the Court of Protection (court appointed deputy)
- an independent mental capacity advocate
- anyone carrying out research approved in accordance with the Act.

But it should be noted that the Joint Committee on the Draft Mental Incapacity Bill reached the following conclusion (the italics are mine):

> 'The position is different with regard to guidance issued to assist non-professional or informal decision makers, such as family members and unpaid carers acting under the *general authority* [to act, to provide care and treatment]. It is essential that family members and paid carers carrying out such responsibilities are provided with appropriate guidance and assistance, both to promote good practice and also to impress upon them the seriousness of their actions and the need to be accountable for them. We accept that it would be inappropriate to impose on them a strict requirement to act in accordance with the Codes of Practice' (Joint Committee on the Draft Mental Incapacity Bill, 2003: para. 232).

### Statutory authority to act reasonably

Chapter 6 of the Code of Practice (referring to section 5 of the MCA) outlines the contextual aspects of the general authority referred to by the Joint Committee, and how the guidance should be followed by different individuals in their respective roles in carrying out any form of treatment or care for a person lacking capacity to make an informed choice about such interventions.

It explicitly confirms the protection that section 5 of the MCA confers on such individuals: within well-defined limits, they are protected from liability for assault or battery in carrying out care. The general authority to act does not imply that another individual can make decisions on behalf of a person lacking capacity; rather, that they are free from liability in carrying out an intervention. The power to make decisions on behalf of someone who lacks capacity is granted through more formal arrangements, via a lasting power of attorney, or a court appointed deputy or by an order of the Court of Protection.

Section 5 does not provide protection for actions that go against the decision of someone authorised to make that decision for a person who lacks capacity. Attorneys and deputies must equally only make decisions that are within the scope of their authority.

The MCA fails to define 'care' and 'treatment', but is intended to clarify aspects of the common law doctrine of necessity in relation to people who lack capacity. The Code is clear that everyday personal care tasks are covered, for example helping someone to wash and dress, preparing food, household cleaning, shopping or helping someone to move home. Medical and nursing treatment are also included, for example carrying out routine medical examinations and tests, taking a person to and from hospital, and giving medication.

If it has been established that the person lacks sufficient capacity to make the decision required and that it is in their best interests, the acts of necessary care may also include paying for goods and services for the person using their own money. The aim is to enable the person to enjoy a standard of living similar to the standard they had before losing capacity by facilitating activities and purchases.

How to judge best interests is discussed in detail in Chapter 3 of this volume, but it is worth emphasising that any act done for, or decision made on behalf of, a person who lacks capacity must be done or made in that person's best interests (MCA: section 1(5)). There are exceptions, which will be explored later in this chapter (e.g. advance decisions and involvement in research), but the Act requires certain steps to be taken. These are set out in the Code of Practice (paras 5.1–5.7) and they include, in broad terms:

- encouraging participation of the individual as far as possible
- identifying all the relevant factors that the individual would have considered
- ascertaining past and present wishes and feelings, beliefs and values.

Although carers can make arrangements for payments to be made on a person's behalf, the Act does not give them access to the person's bank account. Legal authority is necessary for this, via a lasting power of attorney, an order of the Court of Protection or a court appointed deputy (who is likely to be a family member).

Note that a carer cannot make purchases on a person's behalf if this conflicts with decisions made by a person with legal authority over the person's money.

Potentially life-changing decisions also require very careful consideration. A change of home environment may be an entirely appropriate best interests decision, but as the consequences for the person are so significant, the decision cannot be made by informal carers, neighbours or friends. A decision maker (such as the social worker responsible for considering placement in a residential home) would have to discuss best interests principles with relatives or with an independent mental capacity advocate (if no one can be identified to act on the person's behalf).

The Act's principles may apply even if a person states an objection to moving from their home, if they lack capacity to make an informed decision. To fail to act, if the decision is in the person's best interests, could amount to negligence, because failure to conform to a duty of care that left a person in a highly vulnerable position could be seen as contravention of the principles and guidance contained in the Act.

Section 6 of the Act permits restraint, for example in transporting a person to their new home. Section 6(4) defines restraint as 'the use of force or threats to use force, to make someone do something that they are resisting, or restricting a person's freedom of movement, whether they are resisting or not'.

There are limits on the use of restraint. In applying any restraint to a person lacking capacity, the individual taking the action must believe that the restraint is necessary to prevent harm to the person, and the type of restraint used and the time for which it is applied must be proportionate to the likelihood and seriousness of harm. It is permissible, for example, to use proportionate restraint to prevent an elderly person with acute delirium from leaving hospital in the middle of the night, or to stop someone who lacks capacity from crossing a busy road independently when they have no concept of the need for caution.

Indeed, health and social care staff have a common law duty of care outside the provisions of the MCA that requires them to take immediate action to restrain, or remove from a particular environment, a person in their care who lacks capacity, if that individual is presenting with behaviour that is challenging and is a risk to themselves or others, or both.

Section 6 makes it clear that there are limitations to the types of intervention that would be free from liability and that the Act does not confer protection if there is, for example, inappropriate use of restraint or deprivation of liberty. Thus, restraint that includes sedation would be more likely to be defined as deprivation of liberty (which is not permitted under section 5) rather than restriction of a person's freedom (which is permitted under section 5 in clearly defined circumstances). Where the use of restraint strays into the realms of deprivation of liberty is discussed more fully in Chapter 5 of this volume, which considers the Deprivation of Liberty Safeguards.

The European Court of Human Rights has stated that the difference between restricting a person's liberty and depriving them of their liberty is 'one of degree or intensity and not one of nature or substance' (*HL v The United Kingdom*, 2004: para. 89).

Understanding the extent and, moreover, the limits of the duty of care owed, for example, by care providers to individuals who lack capacity is a fundamental tenet of the Mental Capacity Act. In making a distinction between allowing people to put themselves at risk and enabling them to choose to take reasonable risks, a duty of care does not extend to keeping individuals safe from every eventuality.

Inherent in the evaluation of any restraint is respect for the dignity of the individual and for autonomous decision-making, and promotion of overall well-being and self-reliance (King's College London & London School of Economics, 2007). The inappropriate use of restraint is against the law. Restraint can constitute a battery, assault or false imprisonment and can lead to criminal prosecution. The Deprivation of Liberty Safeguards should confer additional protection to vulnerable people and minimise the risk of such practices occurring.

Section 5 of the MCA allows for necessary medical treatment to be carried out, even to the extent of admission to hospital for a person who lacks capacity to make an informed choice and who objects to the proposed treatment or admission. Once again, however, there are limits to the degree of force or restraint that can be imposed.

'Major' healthcare and treatment decisions, in common with decisions about change of residency (as above), require special consideration. Major surgery and 'do not attempt resuscitation' orders would come into this category, unless there is a valid and applicable advance decision to refuse the treatment in question. Special care should be taken in considering the person's best interests. As with residency decisions, an independent mental capacity advocate may need to be consulted if there are no significant carers or relatives.

Final responsibility for a best interests decision lies with the 'decision maker', who is the person proposing the intervention: in the case of medical treatment, the surgeon or physician. Recording the outcome of the best interests assessment is mandatory.

Some treatment decisions are so serious that the Court of Protection has to make them, unless the person has previously set up a lasting power of attorney or an advance decision, although in the case of the latter, advance refusals of life-sustaining treatment must be explicitly recorded in writing.

The Court of Protection must be asked to decide on behalf of someone who lacks capacity in the following situations:

1  The proposed withholding or withdrawal of artificial nutrition and hydration (ANH) from a patient in a persistent vegetative state (PVS).

2  Organ or bone marrow donation by a person who lacks capacity to consent.

3  Medical treatments or procedures that confer direct benefit not on the person but on a third party – the Court might determine that, overall, such an intervention is in the person's best interests through the merit of benefiting a close relation, as in the case of *Re Y (Mental Incapacity: Bone Marrow Transplant)* [1996].

   As section 4(6) of the MCA requires decision makers to consider any factors that the person who lacks capacity would consider if they were able to do so, this might include the effect of the decision on other people: thus, 'best interests' go beyond merely the person's medical interests. In the case of Y, a woman who lacked capacity, the Court decided that it was in her best interests to donate a kidney to her sibling, ruling that the wider benefits to Y, in terms of emotional support from her mother (which might be diminished if her sister's health deteriorated or she were to die) was an important factor in working out her best interests.

4   Non-therapeutic (i.e. contraceptive) sterilisation.

5   Cases where there is a dispute about whether a particular treatment is in a person's best interests. This might include ethical dilemmas concerning untested or innovative treatments, treatments where the risks *v*. benefits are finely balanced, and conflict between professionals and family that cannot be resolved by informal negotiation and discussion.

The giving of urgent treatment without delay to save a person's life is almost always appropriate, unless a valid advance decision to refuse treatment exists, is known to clinical staff and is applicable in the circumstances. In the case of *Marshall v Curry* [1933] the Court held that the removal of a testicle during a surgical procedure for a hernia was necessary, having heard evidence from the surgeon that it was essential to the patient's health and could not have been postponed.

Health and social care staff will be expected to show a higher level of expertise in the areas of capacity assessment and best interests decision-making than, for example, informal carers. Individuals who lack capacity have the same rights as anyone else to pursue a claim in negligence (Code of Practice: para. 6.33). This is analogous to the law of negligence, where professionals are expected to exercise a higher level of care than non-professionals. The MCA does not, however, establish any formal procedure for capacity assessment and there is no statutory form that needs to be completed.

At its heart, the law relating to informed consent is the defence for the professional against a charge of battery in carrying out a particular procedure, i.e. that the patient understands 'in broad terms [...] the nature of the procedure which is intended' (*Chatterson v Gerson*, 1981). There is a difference between understanding in broad terms about a proposed treatment and what information a doctor would reasonably be expected to provide about a proposed treatment (under the law of negligence – *Sidaway v Board of Governors of the Bethlem Royal Hospital*, 1985), meaning that in law there is some conflict about the level of understanding required for a person to be deemed to have capacity.

Nevertheless, the Code of Practice in its guidance on capacity assessment states (at paras 4.44–4.45) that a decision maker who believes a person to lack capacity is required to have reasonable grounds and objective reasons for this view, and to describe the process they took to reach this conclusion.

Readers should refer to Chapters 2 and 3 of this volume for more comprehensive discussion of capacity assessment and best interests decision-making in these areas.

The MCA places the common law authority to make advance decisions to refuse treatment on a statutory footing provided that they are made by a capacitous person over 18 years of age. A valid and applicable advance decision refusing a proposed treatment/intervention must be respected. (Code of Practice: para. 9.1). A doctor would not be protected from liability in carrying out an intervention contrary to that decision (para. 9.2). See pp. 69–71 for more detailed guidance.

# Lasting powers of attorney

The Enduring Powers of Attorney Act 1985 enabled people to grant permission to someone else (the donee, commonly known as the attorney) to manage their property and affairs. A signed but unregistered EPA could be used before a person lost capacity to manage their own affairs, but only if the person gave their consent. Once there were doubts about capacity to manage such affairs independently, the attorney was under an obligation to register the EPA with the Court of Protection.

Such enduring powers of attorney (EPAs) can no longer be made, but those already registered with the Court of Protection remain in force, and any signed by both parties – donor and donee – before 1 October 2007 can still be registered. The Office of the Public Guardian now fulfils this registration role.

The Mental Capacity Act 2005 replaced the enduring power of attorney with the lasting power of attorney (LPA). This introduced provisions for people to choose someone not only to manage their financial affairs (under a property and affairs LPA), but also to make health and welfare decisions (under a personal welfare LPA, also known as a health and welfare LPA) in the event that they lose the capacity, through any 'disorder or disability of mind' that impairs decision-making skills, to make those decisions themselves.

It should be noted that attorneys acting under an EPA do not have a legal duty to have regard to the guidance in the MCA Code of Practice. Attorneys acting under an LPA do.

## General rules governing attorneys under LPAs

An LPA can be created by anyone over the age of 18, provided they have the capacity to do so. Proposed attorneys must carefully consider whether they are prepared for the responsibilities bestowed on them. They must ask themselves whether they have not only the necessary skills to act, but also the desire and time commitment. Section 9(4) of the MCA sets out the requirements for attorneys: they must follow the statutory principles embedded in section 1 of the Act and make decisions in the best interests of the individual (section 4 of the Act). They must also respect any conditions or restrictions that the LPA contains.

Attorneys should refer to Chapter 4 of the Code of Practice when assessing capacity to make particular decisions, following the steps for establishing a 'reasonable belief' that the donor lacks capacity, and also the guidance in Chapter 5 of the Code of Practice in determining best interests.

Attorneys must consider the roles and responsibilities inherent in the authority. Before acting on an LPA, the attorney must, of course, ensure that it is registered with the Office of the Public Guardian. They must take all steps to enable the donor to make the decision in question. They must follow the principles of the MCA and must have regard to the guidance in the Code of Practice.

They have a duty to not take advantage of their position and not benefit themselves but benefit only the donor (fiduciary duty). They must not delegate decisions (unless authorised to do so explicitly in the creation of the LPA), they must respect confidentiality and they must comply with directions of the Court of Protection.

An attorney under an LPA cannot make a will or amend an existing will. If no will exists, an attorney can apply to the Court of Protection for a statutory will (MCA: section 18(1)). The mechanics of the Court's jurisdiction to make wills is contained in Schedule 2 of the MCA.

Attorneys who are not paid should apply the same level/principles of care that they do to their own affairs, but paid attorneys are expected to demonstrate a higher level of care/skills. If a professional attorney (solicitor, accountant) is appointed, they would be expected to comply with their respective professional codes, rules and standards of practice (Code of Practice: para. 7.59).

All attorneys have a duty of care towards the donor, in recognition that the role carries with it a great deal of power (Code of Practice: paras 7.58–7.68).

## Property and financial affairs LPAs

The property and financial affairs LPA effectively transfers authority for making financial and other such decisions to another individual (the attorney/ donee). This enables that individual to make the type of decisions that the donor would have made before they lost capacity. A property and affairs LPA must be registered with the Office of the Public Guardian before it can be used. Unless otherwise stated in the LPA (see next paragraph), the attorney receives the full range of authority relating to property and affairs of the donor, even if the donor retains capacity to make the decisions. This does not remove the authority from a capacitous donor, and the attorney must consult them before making decisions on their behalf.

There is provision within the setting up of a property and affairs LPA that restricts the authority to act to a time when the donor's capacity to make decisions has been lost. It is the donor's responsibility to state who should decide that capacity has been lost. For example, the donor may trust the attorney alone to make the decision, or they may require that their GP or another doctor confirms it in writing.

Note that for as long as they remain competent, donors have the right to override an attorney's decisions and to cancel a property and affairs LPA.

A property and affairs LPA can also be set up when a person no longer has sufficient capacity to manage their affairs, but has sufficient capacity to create an LPA. The approach within the MCA mirrors the case law judgment in *Re K, Re F* [1988], which held that a donor could have capacity to execute an EPA even if they did not have capacity to manage their property and affairs. The judge held that the donor should understand:

> 'first, if such be the terms of the power, that the attorney will be able to assume complete control over the donor's affairs; second, if such be the terms of the power, that the attorney will in general be able to do anything with the donor's property which the donor could have done; third, that the authority will continue if the donor should be or become mentally incapable; fourth, that if he should be or become mentally incapable, the power will be irrevocable without the confirmation of the court.'

If the donor does not restrict the decisions that their property and affairs attorney can make, the attorney's responsibilities might include:

- buying or selling property
- dealing with tax affairs
- paying the mortgage, rent and household expenses
- investing savings
- applying for entitlement to National Health Service continuing care.

The list is extensive and is detailed more comprehensively in the Code of Practice (para. 7.36).

The donor must choose someone who is over 18, is trustworthy, competent and reliable, and not bankrupt at the time of the setting up of the LPA (Code of Practice: paras 7.9–7.13). The attorney must keep accounts and keep the donor's money and property separate from their own.

## Personal welfare (health and welfare) LPAs

A personal welfare LPA (also called a health and welfare LPA) similarly provides authority to another (the attorney/donee) to make certain welfare decisions in the event that a person loses capacity to do so autonomously. The LPA must be registered with the Office of the Public Guardian before it can be used.

A personal welfare LPA can only be used after the donor has lost decision-making capacity, and it extends only to specific decisions for which the individual actually lacks capacity. Such decisions might include: where a person should reside; day-to-day care and dress; to whom they will or will not have access; accessing medical care; consent to medical treatment; applying for confidential documents and personal correspondence; and complaints about care and treatment (Code of Practice: paras 7.21–7.31).

The donor can specify in the LPA any restrictions to the attorney's decision-making authority (e.g. allowing the attorney to make accommodation and social care decisions, but not decisions regarding medical treatment). The attorney cannot consent to or refuse life-sustaining treatment unless the donor has clearly authorised this in the LPA.

Note that treatment for a mental disorder under Part 4 of the Mental Health Act always trumps an LPA or an advance directive, except those treatments regulated by section 58A of the MHA (see 'Excluded decisions', p. 71 below).

## How to create an LPA

Standard forms must be used for each type of LPA. These forms, together with guidance materials, are available from the Office of the Public Guardian. The mechanisms for making, registering and revoking LPAs are also contained in sections 10 and 13 of the MCA and paras 7.6–7.17 of the Code of Practice. Both donor and attorney must be over 18 and the standard form must show the witnessed signatures of the donor and attorney. In addition, a certificate (Part B of the LPA form) must be submitted that confirms that the donor understands the nature and effect of the LPA, that there has been no undue pressure or fraud applied and that there is nothing to stop the LPA being created. This certificate of capacity must be signed by a person who has known the donor for at least 2 years or is a healthcare professional, lawyer, social worker or independent mental capacity advocate. The certificate provider cannot be a family member, the proposed attorney or a relative of the attorney. For property and affairs the attorney could be either a person or a trust corporation, but for personal welfare the attorney must be a named individual.

One or more attorneys can be appointed and separate attorneys can be appointed for the welfare LPA and the property and affairs LPA; they can act alone or together ('jointly and severally'), or always together ('jointly'), and there can be different arrangements for different decisions. Donors can nominate, in advance, replacements in the event of an attorney's death, but attorneys cannot nominate a substitute or successor.

The document itself must also name at least one person (and up to five) who must be notified prior to the registration. These people cannot be any of the attorneys. If the donor wishes no one to be told, two LPA certificate providers must be arranged. This is to ensure that a further person is informed about the application to register the LPA.

As mentioned above, a personal welfare attorney must be a named individual. If a partner or spouse is chosen, dissolution or annulment of the partnership or marriage will mean that the LPA will cease to be valid unless a condition of continuation in such circumstances has been specified in the original document (MCA: section 13(6)).

The fee for registration of an LPA is (at the time of writing) £130. Although a property and affairs LPA can be registered as soon as it is created or when the donor loses capacity to make certain decisions, no action can be taken on the donor's behalf until it has been registered. At the time of writing, the average length of time for registration is 10 weeks from the submission date.

A separate fee is required for each LPA. There are, however, remissions or exemptions from payment of fees based on the donor's financial circumstances (the donor's annual income or receipt of means-tested benefits such as income support, job-seeker's allowance and housing benefit).

The use of a solicitor to assist with the creation and submission of an LPA will, of course, add to costs but is to be recommended, particularly if the donor's circumstances are complicated in any way.

In summary, the following people are involved in the creation of an LPA:

- the donor
- the attorney (donee)
- at least one named person to be notified when the application is made to register the LPA; this individual has the right to object to the registration if they have any doubts about it, thus providing an additional safeguard to the donor
- the certificate provider – a person selected by the donor to complete a Part B in the LPA form, confirming that the donor understands the process and is not under any pressure to create the LPA
- a witness, who signs to confirm that they have witnessed the donor and the attorney/s signing and dating the completed LPA form; a different witness could be used for each signatory.

An attorney cannot make any changes to a completed LPA, as a signed, witnessed and certified LPA is a deed.

Note that each attorney must sign to confirm they have read the explanatory information and understand the duties imposed on them.

# Office of the Public Guardian

The Office of the Public Guardian (OPG) was established in 2007 under the MCA. It supports the Public Guardian in its responsibilities for the registration of EPAs and LPAs and in its supervisory role with respect to court appointed deputies. It is an agency of the Ministry of Justice, and replaced the Public Guardianship Office, which was the administrative arm of the Court of Protection.

As head of the OPG, the Public Guardian has responsibility not only for registering all LPAs, but also for maintaining the register and dealing with any disputes in relation to LPAs, including any complaints about the way attorneys are carrying out their duties.

The OPG also provides information on all aspects of mental capacity to the public, to health and social care professionals, to the legal profession, and to researchers. Furthermore, it has responsibility for policy issues relating to the MCA and to matters of mental capacity in general.

# Court of Protection

The Court of Protection has the same powers, rights, privileges and authority as the High Court in England and Wales. Under the MCA, it can: decide whether a person has capacity to make particular decisions; make declarations (rulings), decisions or orders on financial or welfare matters affecting people who lack capacity; decide whether or not an LPA or EPA is valid; appoint deputies; remove attorneys or deputies who fail to exercise their authority appropriately; and hear cases of objections to the registration of LPAs and EPAs. The Court provides decision-making functions, with the OPG providing regulation and supervision.

In rare instances, the Court of Protection hears cases involving individuals aged under 16; alternatively, it transfers such cases to a court with powers under the Children Act 1989. It can also hear cases of people aged 16 or 17 who lack capacity to make a specific decision, but such cases can also be heard by a family proceedings court.

An application to the Court of Protection to make a particular decision may be necessary when disagreements (e.g. between family members) cannot be resolved, for particularly difficult decisions (e.g. an application by a National Health Service trust to carry out serious medical treatment), and situations where ongoing decisions need to be made about the personal welfare of a person lacking capacity to decide and where there is no other valid authority. The Court's powers to make decisions over personal welfare and property and affairs are defined in the MCA. For personal welfare (MCA: section 17) its powers include:

- deciding where a person should live
- deciding what contact a person can have with other specified individuals
- making an order prohibiting a specified individual from contact with a person
- giving or refusing consent to the carrying out or continuation of a medical treatment.

For property and affairs (MCA: section 18) they include:

- disposition or acquisition of property
- discharge of debts, execution of a will.

Where families disagree, for example about where a person should reside, the Court can make a best interests decision. The Court can also grant an order that has the effect of depriving the person of their liberty, if it is in the person's best interests. If no property and affairs LPA or EPA exists the Court can make a one-off decision, or order, in respect of a person's property and affairs when a particular financial decision needs to made (e.g. to terminate a tenancy agreement, or to make or amend a will).

Sometimes it is not practicable for the Court to make a single declaration or decision, and in such instances a deputy can be appointed (see 'Court appointed deputies', p. 67).

If the person's sole income is from State benefits, an appointee will be more appropriate. This individual (often a relative or friend), appointed by an officer acting on behalf of the Secretary of State, is responsible for all of the person's dealings with the Department for Work and Pensions, and they receive and manage the person's benefits (Department for Work and Pensions, 2011: para. 5050).

Although not covered by the MCA, such appointees are nevertheless expected to conform to the principles of the Act in carrying out their functions.

If a person makes an application to the Court disputing a finding that they lack capacity in relation to a specific decision, that person will always be party to the proceedings of the Court. In all other cases, however, it is at the Court's discretion whether the person is involved personally or represented by an official solicitor appointed by the Court.

In most circumstances, the permission of the Court must be obtained to make any application. The following people, however, have an automatic right to apply to the Court:

- any person who lacks capacity or is alleged to lack capacity to make a specific decision
- the donor or the attorney of an LPA
- a court appointed deputy
- the parents of an allegedly incapacitous person under 18
- a person named in an existing Court order that relates to the application.

In some cases rights of appeal exist, with permission, to higher judges or to the Court of Appeal.

## Court appointed deputies

The OPG and Court of Protection work closely together to protect the interests of those who lack capacity to make decisions for themselves. If there is no LPA (or EPA) for a person who lacks capacity, the Court of Protection may appoint someone to make decisions on that person's behalf. Before the MCA came into effect, such individuals were called receivers and their decision-making powers were restricted to property and affairs. Since 2007, the role of receiver has been replaced with that of court appointed deputy and extended to include health and welfare decisions (although in practice deputies rarely make such decisions).

The duties of court appointed deputies (Code of Practice: paras 8.50–8.68) are subject to the supervision of the Court. Deputies are expected to send periodic reports to the Public Guardian, who also has the authority to investigate complaints made against the exercise of a deputy's authority.

Deputies cannot: prohibit contact with named persons; direct healthcare providers to allow another to take over responsibility; settle or execute a will; exercise any power of consent on behalf of the person; override a decision within the scope of the authority of a donee of an LPA; refuse consent to life-sustaining treatment; and restrain the person (unless four conditions are met, as with LPA holders, and the act is within the scope of authority expressly conferred by the Court) (Code of Practice: paras 8.46–8.54)

An individual (or trust corporation, in the case of property and affairs) applying to the Court to be appointed as a deputy must use the prescribed application form (COP1) and declaration (COP4), and pay certain fees. Family members are most likely to pursue this process. Only the Court can decide who would be the best person to carry out this role, and decide on the extent of any authority bestowed on the deputy, via a deputy order. The deputy must be trustworthy, possess the necessary skills for the role and must follow the principles of the MCA in the same way as holders of an LPA must (Code of Practice: paras 8.40–8.43).

Deputies are appointed under the same principles, and with the same duties, restrictions and responsibilities, as attorneys under LPAs, including that they must be 18 or over, can be appointed to act jointly or severally, albeit that the breadth of the responsibilities and restrictions are determined by the Court of Protection rather than by the donor as in the case of an LPA.

They are expected to act with due skill and care, to respect a fiduciary duty and to refrain from delegating duties, as are attorneys under LPAs, but in addition, deputies must 'indemnify the person against liability to third parties caused by the deputy's negligence'.

Responsibility for supervision of deputies lies with the OPG. In coming to a decision regarding the appointment of a particular deputy, the Court may ask the OPG to obtain a report on the individual, and this may involve the OPG sending a Court of Protection visitor to gather the facts of the case. Once the Court has made an order, the OPG must monitor and supervise the deputy. The OPG decides on the level of supervision required. Anyone who suspects that a deputy is abusing their position should contact the OPG immediately. The OPG may instruct a Court of Protection visitor to visit a deputy to investigate any matter of concern. It can also apply to the Court to cancel a deputy's appointment.

There are supervision fees, which depend on the complexities of the supervision process. At the time of writing, there is a £35 administration fee for minimal supervision (Type 3), and a fee of £320 for light (Type 2), intermediate (Type 2A) or close supervision (Type 1). Under certain circumstances the fees will be waived or will be proportionately lower, depending on the financial circumstances of the donor (not the deputy). Fees can be claimed back from the donor's funds when a deputy seeks to register the documentation.

An application to search the OPG registers for any LPAs, EPAs and court appointed deputies in relation to a particular person is currently free of charge.

If a deputy fails to meet the supervision requirements, the OPG has the power to take the case back to Court, where it will be reviewed and the deputy appointment may be terminated.

Deputies are most commonly appointed for property and affairs. They are rarely required for welfare decisions, and only in the most difficult circumstances, for example where a person's treatment cannot be carried out without the authority of the Court (and it is impractical for the Court to be required to make what is anticipated to be a series of decisions), or where there is no other way of settling a dispute regarding the person's best interests (because of a history of doubts about family members acting in the person's best interests).

## Advance decisions

Aspects of advance decision-making have already been discussed in Chapters 2 and 3, and I will not repeat them here.

The provision for people over 18 (with capacity) to set down in writing, or express verbally, an advance decision to refuse treatment should they lose capacity to make such a decision autonomously in the future was introduced as part of the Mental Capacity Act. It puts on a statutory footing the former common law obligation of healthcare professionals to respect such advance decisions provided that the decision to be made was valid and applicable.

A valid and applicable advance decision has the same force as a contemporaneous decision. An advance decision cannot require a specific treatment to be provided, nor does it permit anything that would be contrary to the criminal law relating to homicide, euthanasia and assisted suicide (MCA: section 62; Code of Practice: para. 9.6). Rather, it is the competent refusal of consent to a particular treatment and, in line with this, will not apply where consent is not necessary (under section 4 of the Mental Health Act).

Treatment includes 'diagnostic or other procedures' (MCA: section 64) but refers essentially to treatment in a medical context. Thus, a person cannot make an advance refusal, for example, to care home placement.

The MCA allows the person to refuse all treatment and the Code of Practice confirms that the advance decision 'must state precisely what treatment is to be refused – a statement giving a general desire not to be treated is not enough' (Code of Practice: para. 9.11).

An advance decision takes precedence over any consent given by an attorney under an LPA or by a court appointed deputy. The Court of Protection has the authority to determine the validity or applicability of an advance decision, but it cannot override a valid and applicable decision.

An advance decision to refuse life-sustaining treatment must be recorded in writing, be signed and witnessed, and it must state explicitly an understanding of the consequences of the refusal.

Health professionals can act against an advance decision if they have reason to believe that it is not valid or applicable in the circumstances at hand, or if they are unaware of its existence. In such circumstances, they will be immune from liability. They must, however, pay due respect to the general expression of the wishes contained in an advance decision when making a best interests decision. That is, they must take account of all the factors that the person would have taken into consideration in making the decision at hand, which may be expressed even if the actual advance decision is not applicable in the circumstances.

Doubts about a person's capacity to make an advance decision can render it invalid. Validity may also be questionable if the person later acts in a manner that is clearly contrary to the wishes expressed in the advance decision document. Equally, unless the advance decision specifies exactly what treatment is to be refused, and in what circumstances, it may not be applicable.

Changes in the individual's personal life or a novel treatment not anticipated in the advance decision might be relevant to its application. This is particularly pertinent if a long time has elapsed since its creation and a new treatment has become available that might have materially affected the person's decision. Equally, if a person behaves in a way clearly inconsistent with the advance decision, then there are grounds to question its applicability, for example if they consent to a blood transfusion after making an advance decision to refuse the intervention (*HE v a Hospital NHS Trust*, 2003).

Professionals are protected from liability in providing treatment if they have genuine doubts about the validity or applicability of an advance decision, provided that they act in the person's best interests (MCA: section 26; Code of Practice: paras 9.57–9.60). Thus, they are also protected when providing life-sustaining treatment or carrying out any act reasonably believed to be necessary to protect life or prevent serious deterioration in a person's condition (the doctrine of necessity) while a decision regarding the existence, validity or applicability of an advance decision is being sought from the Court.

The person making the advance decision must sign the document or nominate someone to sign on their behalf. Alternatively, it can be written down on their behalf and a witness must sign it in the presence of the person making the decision. Witnessing the signature of a person who has made a written advance decision (or the signature of someone nominated to sign on their behalf) is essential if the person is refusing life-sustaining interventions. It is merely the signature that is witnessed: the witness is not certifying that the person has capacity to make the decision. However, a professional may act as both witness and assessor of capacity, in which case a record of the capacity assessment must be made.

Some people seek medical and/or legal advice about making advance decisions. Verbal advance decisions can be recorded, for example, in case records by healthcare professionals. It is the responsibility of the person making an advance decision to alert necessary individuals, including healthcare professionals and family members, of its existence (Code of Practice: para. 9.38).

If a verbal advance decision is made during a clinical encounter, the person's healthcare record should include: a note that the decision should apply in the event of future incapacity; a clear note of the decision, including the specific treatment to be refused and circumstances of refusal; details of anyone else present during the interview and their role in the interview process; and whether they heard the decision and/or took part in it.

An advance decision cannot involve the refusal of certain basic care, for example warmth, shelter and the offer of food and fluid by mouth. These should continue to be provided under the general authority to act in the person's best interests. However, an advance decision can refuse artificial nutrition and hydration (MCA: section 5; Code of Practice: para. 9.28).

Advance decisions should be regularly reviewed by the person who made them and updated as necessary; they can be cancelled at any time.

Best interests principles do not apply in carrying out an advance decision, as the decision reflects previously expressed autonomous decision-making. As already mentioned, advance decisions made before the MCA came into force may still be valid and applicable under the common law obligation.

A valid and applicable advance decision to refuse treatment overrules any pre-existing personal welfare LPA, so the LPA attorney cannot give consent to treatment that has been refused in the advance decision. However, an LPA made after an advance decision will render the advance decision invalid, if it provides authority to the attorney to make decisions about the same treatment (Code of Practice: paras 9.33–9.34).

Generally, an advance decision to refuse treatment for a mental disorder can be overruled if the person is detained under the Mental Health Act, when treatment can be given compulsorily under Part 4 of the Act (MCA Code of Practice: para. 9.37). The exception, under section 58A, is that advance refusal of electroconvulsive therapy (ECT) must be respected.

## Excluded decisions

The MCA does not permit certain decisions to be made on behalf of a person who lacks capacity to consent. These include family relationship decisions such as consenting to: marriage or civil partnership; sexual relations; a decree of divorce or dissolution of a civil partnership on the basis of 2 years' separation; a child being placed in adoption; an adoption order; an action under the Human Fertilisation and Embryology Act.

The following are equally expressly not authorised by the MCA: giving medical treatment for a mental disorder and consenting on behalf of a person being given medical treatment for a mental disorder, if treatment is already regulated by Part 4 of the Mental Health Act.

## Voting rights

The MCA does not permit voting on behalf of an individual lacking capacity, at an election for any public office or at a referendum.

# Research

The MCA does not define research, but it conforms to the definition given in the *Research Governance Framework for Health and Social Care*: 'Research can be defined as the attempt to derive generalisable new knowledge by addressing clearly defined questions with systematic and rigorous methods' (Department of Health, 2005: para. 1.10). Research projects can demonstrate how effective and safe a novel treatment is and can add evidence to promote the efficacy and/or safety of one mode of treatment over another.

The emotive subject of conducting research on individuals who lack capacity to give informed consent to the process has been formally debated, and ultimately sanctioned, in recent years. Before the MCA came into effect, there were no formal restrictions relating to carrying out research involving incapacitous adults, with the result that studies were conducted with no safeguards as to its appropriateness. However, an outright ban was undesirable, as it would effectively have halted advancements in the knowledge of the conditions causing incapacity, so an approach involving the imposition of structures and limitations was developed.

The MCA Code of Practice provides for people without capacity to benefit from participation in properly conducted research, with provision also for strict protective safeguards.

The MCA applies to all research that is intrusive, i.e. that would be unlawful without the informed consent of the individual. The Act does not apply to research involving clinical trials of new drugs, as when it was drawn up these were already covered by the Medicines for Human Use (Clinical Trials) Regulations 2004. These regulations were amended in 2006 to enable consistency with the Mental Capacity Act in so far as they relate to emergency research conducted on incapacitous patients (Secretary of State, 2006).

The MCA provides statutory guidance about the rights and responsibilities of all concerned in this area. It sets out: the criteria governing when it is permissible to carry out research on a person who lacks capacity; provisions on obtaining ethical approval, respecting the wishes of the research participants, and engaging with participants and their relatives/carers; the responsibilities of the researchers; and how the new legislation applies to research begun before the Act came into force.

Notably, the sections concerning research (sections 30–34) do not refer to a best interests test. They do, however, introduce other thresholds, in particular that the research must either have the potential to benefit the person taking part ( therapeutic intervention) or be intended to provide knowledge of the cause of, or treatments for, the condition, or of care for people with the same or a similar condition (non-therapeutic intervention).

Potential benefits for recruited participants include the development of more effective treatments, improving the quality of health and social care, discovering the causes of the condition and reducing risks to the individuals of harm and discrimination. Benefits may not be immediately experienced on completion of the project.

Because of the distinction between research that may benefit the participant and that in which the participant is in effect playing an altruistic role, the MCA imposes different thresholds of 'burden' allowed in the two cases. In the first case, the burden on the participant should not be disproportionate to the benefit to them; in the second, research must carry virtually no burden of participation (MCA: section 33). In practice, these are difficult judgements to make, as what is burdensome to one person might not be to another.

In addition to the requirement that research on individuals who lack capacity to give informed consent be designed to help understand or treat their condition, it is also required that the research cannot be carried out as effectively on individuals who can give informed consent.

Note that in certain circumstances, no consent is needed to lawfully involve a person in research, regardless of whether they are able to give informed consent or not. This applies in relation to, for example, anonymised data or anonymised tissue taken from a living person.

Responsibility for meeting the Act's requirements lies with the researchers and the 'appropriate body' as defined in regulations. In England, such regulations are set by the Secretary of State and the 'body' must be a research ethics committee recognised by the Secretary of State. In Wales, the regulations are set by the National Assembly for Wales and the 'body' must be a research ethics committee recognised by the Welsh Assembly Government.

Research approval must be obtained from the appropriate body, and researchers must consider the views of the relatives and carers, must treat the individual participant's interests as more important than the interests of science and society, and moreover, regardless of the participant's incapacity, must respect any objections that the individual makes during the research project (Code of Practice: para. 11.20).

Carers or family members interested in the person's well-being (and willing to participate) must be consulted before any potential participant is recruited. This 'consultee' must be able to withdraw the individual at any time before or during the research process. If, however, the consultee wishes for the person to be removed from the study after it has begun, the researchers may decide against withdrawal if they believe that it would cause significant risk to the person's health, for example if the person is receiving treatment as part of the research. The researchers may decide to continue with the research while this risk continues to exist but they should stop any parts of the study that are not related to the risk (Code of Practice: para. 11.28).

The person must be removed from the study if they show any evidence of distress, or if any of the Act's requirements are no longer met.

The consultee cannot be a professional or paid carer, but can be an attorney authorised under a registered LPA or a deputy appointed by the Court of Protection, as long as they are not acting in a professional or paid capacity.

If no one is easily identifiable as a consultee, the researcher must nominate a person (not involved in the research project) to fulfil the role, following guidance from the Secretary of State for England or the National Assembly for Wales.

Further safeguards for researchers are discussed more fully in the Act and its Code of Practice.

Special rules apply where a person who lacks capacity may be receiving, or is about to receive, emergency treatment and researchers want to include them in a research project. In such circumstances, if a researcher thinks it necessary to take urgent action for the purposes of the research and it is not practicable to consult someone about it, they can only take action if they get agreement from a registered medical practitioner who is not involved in the research project (to avoid conflict of interest) or they follow a procedure that the 'appropriate body' agreed to at the approval stage of the project.

This ability to waive consultation applies only for as long as the situation remains an emergency. It applies only to research into emergency situations, not in situations where a practitioner merely wants to act quickly in a clinical encounter.

The MCA allows the removal of tissue from the body of a person who lacks capacity to give informed consent to its removal, if the procedure is in the person's best interests.

Note that the Human Tissue Act 2004 has different rules for individuals lacking capacity from those that apply to individuals who retain capacity to consent and, additionally, there are specific rules that apply to research begun or approved before 1 October 2007.

## Independent mental capacity advocates

An independent mental capacity advocate (IMCA) is required for a person lacking capacity if the person has no family or friends that it would be appropriate to consult and the decision involves accommodation, or serious medical treatment or a vulnerable adult investigation.

The IMCA arrangements have regard to the principle that (insofar as is practicable) people should be represented and supported by an individual who is independent of anyone responsible for the act or decision in question.

There will be no IMCA appointment, therefore, if the person in question has nominated (in whatever manner) someone that they would like to be consulted in matters affecting their interests, or if they have already granted an LPA or have a court appointed deputy who continues to act on their behalf.

An IMCA is required for 'serious medical treatment', including the giving of new treatment and the stopping or withholding of current treatment, in circumstances where the proposed treatment is finely balanced in terms of its benefits to the person and the burdens and risks it imposes on them. In addition, where there is a choice of treatments, balanced equally in terms of risks and benefits, or where treatment will involve serious consequences for the patient, an IMCA must be consulted. Examples might include cancer treatment, kidney dialysis, insertion of a percutaneous endoscopic gastrostomy (PEG) feeding tube and a review of a 'do not attempt resuscitation' order. The IMCA requirement does not apply to treatment under Part 4 of the Mental Health Act or to treatment provided in an emergency.

Note that ECT might count as serious medical treatment (Code of Practice: para. 10.45). However, as with all 'serious medical treatment', criteria allow for a degree of discretion to be exercised by the treating clinician as to the characteristics of any proposed therapeutic intervention (Code of Practice: para. 10.45). Neurosurgery, amputations, withholding or withdrawing of artificial nutrition or hydration are all 'serious', albeit the last would require a Court judgment, for which the IMCA would apply through an official solicitor.

The IMCA service does not replace general advocacy services; nor do IMCAs assess capacity or act as best interests decision makers. The IMCA interviews the person, accesses the relevant case records and submits a report to the decision maker. The decision maker must take this report into account.

The role of the IMCA is to provide independent safeguards for people who lack capacity to make certain decisions. They represent the person in discussions about what constitutes best interests, providing information that helps to determine these by ascertaining the person's values, beliefs, wishes and feelings, and raising questions or challenges where they believe certain decisions appear not to conform to best interests principles. They can raise such questions with the Court of Protection. Independent mental capacity advocates have no role for persons detained under the Mental Health Act, except in rare circumstances.

# Neglect

The MCA created an offence of ill-treatment or neglect of an individual lacking capacity by someone who has the care of the person, is their attorney under an LPA or is a court appointed deputy (MCA: section 44).

The elements of ill-treatment were articulated in the case of *R v Newington* (1990). Interpretation of the judgment concludes that the definition is broad enough to include neglect in the sense of inadequate heating, provision of inadequate food, use of verbal aggression and bullying (Gunn, 1990), but there is little guidance on the definition of neglect except as 'a particular state of mind' (*R v Newington*, 1990).

Penalties range from a fine to a sentence of imprisonment of up to 5 years, or both.

## Conclusion

The Mental Capacity Act essentially provides a mechanism by which decisions may be made, and legal relations entered into, on behalf of a person who lacks capacity. It gives the legal framework within which care and treatment may be provided, contracts entered into, wills drafted, and financial, property and some other legal decisions made on behalf of individuals who lack capacity (Bartlett, 2008). It is designed, despite its complexities, as an enabling piece of legislation to protect autonomous decision-making where possible and to ensure that there are adequate safeguards to protect the health and well-being of some of the most vulnerable members of our society.

For those of us who work on a daily basis with individuals who lack capacity to make certain types of decision (and their carers), such terms as best interests, lasting power of attorney, advance decision-making and IMCA have become part of our ordinary language. But the true measure of the success of the legislation to fully deliver what it set out to achieve remains to be seen over time.

## References

Bartlett, P. (2008) *Blackstone's Guide to the Mental Capacity Act 2005* (2nd edn). Oxford University Press.

Department for Constitutional Affairs (2007) *Mental Capacity Act 2005: Code of Practice.* TSO (The Stationery Office).

Department for Work and Pensions (2011) *Agents, Appointees, Attorneys and Deputies Guide (AAADG): September 2011 Amendment Package.* DWP.

Department of Health (2005) *Research Governance Framework for Health and Social Care* (2nd edn). Central Office of Information.

Gunn, M. (1990) Casenote on *R v Newington. Journal of Forensic Psychiatry*, **360**, 361.

Joint Committee on the Draft Mental Incapacity Bill (2003) *Draft Mental Incapacity Bill: Session 2002–03* (vol. 1) (HL Paper 189-I; HC 1083-I). TSO (The Stationery Office).

King's College London & London School of Economics (2007) *Dementia UK: A Report to the Alzheimer's Society on the Prevalence and Economic Costs of Dementia in the UK, Produced by King's College London and the London School of Economics.* Alzheimer's Society.

Secretary of State (2006) *Statutory Instruments 2006 No. 1928: The Medicines for Human Use (Clinical Trials) Amendment (No. 2) Regulations 2006.* TSO (The Stationery Office).

## Case law

*CC v KK and STCC* [2012] 2136 EWHC (COP).

*Chatterson v Gerson* [1981] QB 432 443.

*HE v a Hospital NHS Trust* [2003] EWHC 1017.

*HL v The United Kingdom* [2004] ECHR 720.

*Marshall v Curry* [1933] 3 DLR 260.

*Re K, Re F* [1988] 1 All ER 358.

*Re Y (Mental Incapacity: Bone Marrow Transplant)* [1996] 2 FLR 787.

*R v Newington* (1990) 91 Cr App R 247.

*Sidaway v Board of Governors of the Bethlem Royal Hospital* [1985] AC 871.

# CHAPTER 5

# The Deprivation of Liberty Safeguards

Susan F. Welsh and Amanda Keeling

In terms of their introduction to the statute book, the Deprivation of Liberty Safeguards (DoLS) were created as an amendment to the Mental Capacity Act 2005 through the vehicle of revision of the Mental Health Act 1983 in 2007. They came into statutory force on 1 April 2009 in England and Wales. The legislation puts in place a procedure through which adults over the age of 18, who are shown to lack capacity to decide on their care and treatment, can be deprived of their liberty in a hospital or care home.

The purpose of the safeguards was to deal with an issue highlighted in litigation by Mr HL that concluded in the European Court of Human Rights. This issue, which became known as the Bournewood gap, concerns the rights of individuals whom it has not been considered necessary to detain under sections 2 or 3 of the MHA, but who are in hospital as informal patients without having consented to such admission.

The essence of Mr HL's claim was that he had been unlawfully detained in hospital without the use of the Mental Health Act (MHA). The counterclaim was that he was an uncomplaining man, who was not capable of making decisions and who was lawfully present in hospital by virtue of section 131 of the MHA, which provides for informal admission, and it was felt that the 'doctrine of necessity' justified the treatment and restrictions imposed on him by Bournewood Hospital. The European Court found in favour of Mr HL because it took the view that there was a breach of Article 5 of the European Convention on Human Rights, which is part of English law by virtue of the Human Rights Act 1998 (*HL v The United Kingdom*, 2004). Article 5(1) provides that: 'Everyone has the right to liberty and security of the person. No one shall be deprived of his liberty save in the following cases and *in accordance with a procedure prescribed by law*'. The cases listed include: 'the *lawful detention* of persons for the prevention of the spreading of infectious disease, of *persons of unsound mind*, alcoholics or drug addicts, or vagrants' [italics added].

Article 5 applied because Mr HL was deprived of his liberty owing to the fact that healthcare professionals were able to exercise 'full control of the liberty and treatment of a vulnerable incapacitated individual solely on the basis of their own clinical assessments completed as and when they considered fit' (*HL v The United Kingdom*, 2004). The Court found that there was a lack of any procedural rules by which the admission and detention of compliant, incapacitated (incapacitous) patients was conducted. There was no formalised admission procedure determining who could propose admission, for what reasons and on the basis of what kind of medical assessment. There was no requirement to establish an exact purpose for the admission and no time limits attached to it. There was no provision for a patient's representative to make any objections or applications against the detention on their behalf. This meant that not only was there a breach of Article 5(1), but also Article 5(4), which provides that: 'Everyone who is deprived of his liberty by arrest or detention shall be entitled to take proceedings by which the lawfulness of his detention shall be decided speedily by a court and his release ordered if the detention is not lawful'.

Following this decision, it was clear that the position of incapable, non-complaining patients resident in hospital or other care accommodation needed to be addressed. A number of options were explored, including amending the current mental health legislation to incorporate the necessary safeguards, i.e. to extend the use of detention under the Mental Health Act as amended in 2007 or to extend the use of guardianship under the Act. To these was added a third option, that of protective care. It was the latter that was preferred in the consultation exercise run by the Department of Health (Department of Health, 2005). The option of providing protection for vulnerable adults through the Mental Capacity Act (MCA) rather than mental health legislation was thought to be justified on the basis of three key factors. First, it would be appropriate to utilise the structure for decision-making in the best interests of the incapable adult; second, usage of the MHA would extend the perceived stigma caused by that legislation to a broader group of people; and third, use of the MHA would be a disproportionate response as it was not the least restrictive option. The protective care option became the Deprivation of Liberty Safeguards. Although this approach might be regrettable (a better option might have been to require greater use of either the MHA or the MCA), it is the option that has been adopted, and sense has to be made of the legislation.

## Who may be subject to DoLS?

Those, in England and Wales, who may be made subject to DoLS:

- must be over 18
- must have a mental disorder, which includes significant intellectual disability (learning disability), dementia and certain neurological disorders
- must lack capacity to consent to their care and treatment arrangements
- must be in a situation in which those arrangements involve a deprivation of liberty but are necessary to protect them from harm
- must be in a situation in which use of the MHA is not more appropriate.

For people falling outside these provisions, there are routes for challenging the position in which they find themselves. For people under 18, the child protection legislation applies as it applies to any other young person or child. Where someone is in their own home, the standard provisions of the MCA apply and, as the reach of that legislation is very broad, any concerns can be raised with the Court of Protection.

# What constitutes deprivation of liberty?

As the name implies, the key concept in the DoLS is the deprivation of liberty, as it is only when such a deprivation arises that these particular, extra safeguards come into play. Determining whether there is a deprivation of liberty is not simple. This is partly because the choice has been to use a concept that exists within the European Convention on Human Rights, and so its meaning can only be determined by reference to its use in that context and its developing meaning as determined by the courts, most significantly, the European Court of Human Rights.

The European Court of Human Rights has consistently held that deprivation of liberty should be considered in the 'classic' sense of physical liberty, which is more than just a restriction on freedom of movement (*Engel & Others v The Netherlands*, 1976: para. 58). In deciding whether there is a deprivation of liberty, it is the concrete situation that must be considered. This means the real situation, taking into account a range of criteria, including the type, duration, effects and manner of implementation of the measure in question (*Guzzardi v Italy*, 1980: para. 92). For an infringement of liberty to amount to a deprivation is a question of the 'degree and intensity, not nature or substance' of the restriction (*Guzzardi v Italy*, 1980: para. 93). So, deprivation of liberty can apply to anything that limits freedom of movement, but it only amounts to a deprivation of liberty if the degree and intensity of the infringement are sufficient to warrant regarding it as a deprivation rather than a restriction on liberty, which itself would involve a breach of the Convention but of a different and lesser right.

To help determine whether the infringement is sufficiently serious to warrant being described as a breach of one of the key Articles of the Convention, further consideration of the case law is required. The first relevant step was taken in *JE v DE and Surrey County Council* [2006], a case pre-dating the introduction of the DoLS. On the basis of European case law, and specifically the opinion of the court in *Storck v Germany* (2005), Justice Munby set out a three-part test for deprivation of liberty:

1    an objective element: the person is confined in a particular restricted place for a not negligible length of time
2    a subjective element: the person is not able to, or has not, validly consented
3    the deprivation of liberty is imputable to the State.

In the context of adults lacking capacity whose care is funded by the State, parts two and three are relatively easy to ascertain. It is the objective element in part one that provides the challenge in determining whether a deprivation of liberty is occurring.

In applying his test to the facts, Justice Munby devised what appeared to be a relatively simple test: deprivation of liberty occurred when the individual was prevented from 'leaving in the sense of removing himself permanently in order to live where and with whom he chooses' (*JE v DE*, 2006: para. 115).

The Joint Committee on Human Rights suggested that this be used as a statutory definition in the DoLS legislation and, despite the rejection of the proposal by the government of the day, which resisted such a definition, it was used as the main approach by the courts in several early cases (*Dorset CC v EH*, 2009; *G v E (By his litigation friend the Official Solicitor)*, 2010). Recent cases have, however, moved to a much more nuanced, and less narrow, approach to deprivation of liberty.

The more recent case law can be seen to classify three particular factors as being of relevance when considering deprivation of liberty:

- objection
- context/setting
- family contact.

These factors had been evolving through the case law, and were confirmed as relevant in 2011 by Lord Justice Wilson's leading judgment in *P and Q v Surrey County Council* [2011]. It is therefore suggested that this approach would be a proper starting point for determining whether a deprivation of liberty exists in any particular situation.

## Objection

The relevance of the individual's objection to their situation has long been a subject for discussion when considering whether there is a deprivation of liberty. Several cases have placed a great deal of weight on the person's happiness in their surroundings in finding there to be no deprivation of liberty (e.g. *LLBC v TG*, 2007; *Surrey County Council v CA & LA & MIG & MEG*, 2010, commonly known as *MIG and MEG*). However, the courts have not always been consistent on this point, with the apparent happiness in her surroundings not ameliorating her deprivation of liberty in *BB v AM* (2010). Conversely, the presence of an objection was held to be of significant importance in *JE v DE* in establishing a deprivation of liberty.

The point has recently received some clarification in the appeal of *MIG and MEG*, renamed as *P and Q v Surrey County Council* [2011] in the Court of Appeal. In his judgment, Lord Justice Wilson declared that happiness should not be relevant in determining whether a deprivation of liberty exists. Simply because a person is happy does not mean they cannot be objectively deprived of their liberty. However, Lord Justice Wilson decided that objection is a relevant factor, insofar as the consequences of an objection are likely to be conflict and increased restraint and use of force. Objection should therefore be an indicator of a greater likelihood of a deprivation of liberty.

In a hospital setting, Justice Charles in *GJ v The Foundation Trust & Others* [2009] suggested that an objection would lead to detention under the MHA. So, there may be an issue still to be resolved, which is whether the setting determines the role of objection and the consequence that flows from it. Of course, it is important to recall that the original objective of the DoLS was to provide protection for a compliant, or non-objecting, incapable man.

## Context/setting

The relevance of the setting in determining a deprivation of liberty was first discussed pre-DoLS in *LLBC v TG* (2007), where it was recognised that the applicant lived in an 'ordinary care home where ordinary restrictions applied' and so no deprivation of liberty was found. However, *LLBC v TG* was decided around the same time as *JE v DE*, which took an analysis closer to that of the European Court, examining freedom to leave and the level of control exercised over the person's movements, and this became the dominant method of determining deprivation of liberty. Nevertheless, despite the European Court continuing with this analysis (see the recent judgments in *Stanev v Bulgaria* [2012], *DD v Lithuania* [2012] and *Kedzior v Poland* [2012]), the English courts have more recently reverted to the approach taken in *LLBC v TG* (see *MIG & MEG* above, and *Re A (Adult); Re C (Child); A Local Authority v A*, 2010, known as *Re A and Re C*).

There has been some clarification in Lord Justice Wilson's judgment in *P and Q v Surrey County Council* [2011]. When the case was first heard (as *Surrey County Council v CA & LA & MIG & MEG*, 2010), in a judgment which caused some consternation at the time, Justice Parker found that there was no deprivation of liberty. Greatly persuaded by the idea that many of the limitations on P and Q's freedoms were dictated by their own cognitive limitations, it was permissible to look at the reasons why restrictions on an individual were in place. On appeal, Lord Justice Wilson decided that it was incorrect to look at the reasons or purpose behind any restrictions on liberty, but reframed Justice Parker's judgment as stressing the relative normality of the living arrangements. He decided that, while Justice Parker was misguided to focus on the reasons, she was correct to note that P (MIG) and Q (MEG) were being cared for in a home. What must be considered is not the purpose of the restrictions, but whether the setting, and the restrictions inherent in that setting, still allow the individual to live the most normal life possible. Citing Lord Justice Munby's earlier judgment in *Re A and Re C*, he stated that where the individual resides is an important factor in determining deprivation of liberty. But assessing the normality of the individual's life requires an evaluation beyond just residency. One must consider other aspects, such as social contact, school or college attendance in the case of young adults or children, or other occupations in the case of older adults.

This 'normality' approach appears to be helpful. It means that the more close to a normal life the individual is allowed to lead, the less likely is it that there is a deprivation of liberty. Some restrictions on liberty occur in all our lives, for example most of us sleep at home with the outside doors locked, most of us expect to tell someone with whom we are living where we are going and when we will be back, most of us are expected to engage in certain activity each and every day, and this is activity in which we initially chose to be engaged. So the more this normality is not apparent, the more likely it is that there is a deprivation of liberty.

However, this approach must be considered with caution. In *Cheshire West and Chester Council v P* [2011], Lord Justice Munby declared that a suitable comparator must be found for assessing the normality of the life of the individual, and that it was inappropriate to compare their life to the life they would have had, had they not been disabled. Despite the huge amount of restriction on his daily life, P was not found to be deprived of his liberty. This approach to normality must be continued with caution, and perhaps requires a reassessment of the aim of the DoLS. They were brought in to provide safeguards for a group who do not have a voice, and to monitor the restrictions on their lives to ensure that these are necessary and proportionate. The danger of steering too far down the 'normality' route is that the constant monitoring of restrictive practice will disappear, and the only people for whom the safeguards will be available will be those who experience bad practice and overly excessive restriction bordering on abusive. At the time of writing, both *Cheshire West* and *P and Q* have been given leave to appeal by the Supreme Court. However, the joined appeals of *Cheshire West* and *P and Q* will not be heard until the latter part of 2013, with a judgment unlikely before the end of the year at the earliest.

The European Court of Human Rights has had cause to consider deprivation of liberty since these cases and there is, as indicated by Justice Baker (in *CC v KK and STCC*, 2012), a mismatch between the approach taken by the English Court of Appeal in *Cheshire West* and by Strasbourg. The terms of section 64(5) of the MCA link the definition of a deprivation of liberty for the purposes of the Act to Article 5(1) of the European Convention on Human Rights, meaning that linkage of the MCA is to the Article as interpreted by the Strasbourg Court rather than the English Court. Any discrepancy between the respective jurisdictions makes it difficult to be sure what does or does not constitute deprivation of liberty. Justice Baker stated (in *CC v KK and STCC*, 2012): 'the decision in Cheshire West [...] has been the subject of academic criticism on the grounds that, insofar as it may permit some people to be denied a declaration of deprivation of liberty in circumstances where others would be entitled to such a declaration, it may be discriminatory'. Pending the Supreme Court Appeal therefore, Justice Baker held that 'the right course is to have regard to the purpose for a decision as part of the overall circumstances and context but to focus on the concrete situation in determining whether the objective element is satisfied'. In that particular case, determining whether or not there was a deprivation of liberty, factors that included the measure of control over the individual's (KK's) movements, and her objections, were weighed against factors that included the lack of sedation, lack of restraint, lack of restrictions on contacts with other people, lack of loss of significant personal autonomy, and the 'relative normality' of being in a nursing home and spending time visiting her own home. Her circumstances were felt not to constitute a breach of her rights under Article 5.

It is noteworthy also that the Scottish Law Commission has recently published a discussion paper on adults with incapacity which presents provisional views on options for the Scottish Government to adopt a regime to close the Bournewood gap there (Scottish Law Commission, 2012). Its conclusion is that Scotland should seek to enact a statutory definition of what constitutes (and does not constitute) a deprivation of liberty.

## Mental health settings

The comments made by Lord Justice Wilson regarding normality are very important for mental health settings. Institutional environments provide a wide spectrum of normality, from 'the small children's home or nursing home [to] a hospital designed for compulsory detentions like Bournewood' *(P and Q v Surrey County Council*, 2011). The suggestion in this statement is that, within mental health settings, life is 'abnormal' and that admission to such a setting generally constitutes a deprivation of liberty. This was the interpretation of the Department of Health and, following the judgment, they issued this statement:

> 'Mental health settings are different. [To admit someone without using the MHA] they will need to demonstrate that the regime for those not detained under the [MHA] is distinct and different to the regime of those detained under the MHA. Otherwise, a person who lacks capacity to consent for himself, even when they are not objecting [...] is likely to be deprived of his liberty simply by being in that setting. The Deprivation of Liberty Safeguards will need to be applied in those circumstances even when the person is not objecting' (Department of Health, 2011).

The Department of Health suggests that an environment where compulsory detention and treatment are required cannot be 'normal', and therefore will always result in a deprivation of liberty. This interpretation must be followed with some care, as Lord Justice Wilson was endeavouring to introduce a single standard that could be applied in any setting – and singling out mental health settings risks muddying the waters once again. A formal setting does not necessarily equate to a deprivation of liberty, and some formal settings may be relatively close to normal. However, the more restrictive the environment, the more likely there will be a deprivation of liberty, and what is crucial in the Department of Health's interpretation is the difference in regime for those who are not detained. The less difference there is between the regime for a patient detained under the MHA and that for a patient not detained, the more likely it is that there will be a deprivation of liberty.

## Family contact

The extent and nature of family contact was an important issue in *HL v The United Kingdom* [2004] and *Storck v Germany* (2005), and over time it has become more influential in English DoLS cases. Restrictions on family contact have contributed to findings of a deprivation of liberty in several cases, including *G v E* [2010] and *A Primary Care Trust v P & Others* [2009]. Good family contact was a persuasive factor in the finding of no deprivation of liberty in *LLBC v TG* [2007].

The issue has been more recently highlighted in the case of Mark and Steven Neary (*London Borough of Hillingdon v Neary & Another*, 2011), where the matter of family contact was the most prominent reason for the finding of a deprivation of liberty. Steven Neary, a young man with autism and other complex care needs, lived at home with his father, Mark. While Steven was in a care home for a period of respite care, the local authority decided that Mark was no longer able to meet Steven's care needs and that he should remain in the care home after the end of the respite period. In his judgment, Justice Peter Jackson found that, in keeping Steven away from his home and father, there had been a deprivation of liberty (and further that that deprivation was unlawful because of the way in which it had been enacted). In addition, this contributed to a finding of a breach of Article 8 of the European Convention on Human Rights, the right to family and private life. Article 8 is underused by both the domestic and European courts in cases concerning deprivation of liberty, but should be considered a more useful tool, and the approach taken by the court in the case of Neary is heartening in this respect. It suggests that those working with adults who lack capacity should consider issues of family life to be just as important as factors such as supervision, control and locked doors.

## Conclusion

Despite several high-profile cases, the situation for what constitutes a deprivation of liberty is still not clear and authorities may find themselves 'placed in an invidious position when seeking to avoid claims for breaches of section 5(1) [of the Human Rights Act] on the one hand, and accusations of failure to protect the vulnerable or excessive or inappropriate use of the MHA on the other' (Morris & Ruck Keene, 2007: p. 9).

The best guidance for those working in restrictive environments is to consider the importance of promoting the following principles:

- maximisation of liberty and autonomy
- person-centred care
- involvement of family and friends
- minimisation of restrictions, and constant comparison with the MHA regime
- frequent review of the care plan.

What ultimately amounts to a deprivation of liberty is a legal question and only the courts can determine the law. What clinicians and authorities must endeavour to do is to gather all the relevant information and reach a decision applying the appropriate principles, insofar as they can be determined. Going to court may be necessary to resolve difficult issues, and a decision of the court can be relied on to determine such issues.

# Eligibility for DoLS – the link with the MHA

The aim of the DoLS was to provide not an 'alternative' framework for detention to the MHA, but rather a parallel system which bridged the Bournewood gap (see p. 78).

Schedule 1A to the MCA gives the procedure for determining eligibility for the DoLS. This procedure and its interpretation have been set out by Justice Charles in *GJ v The Foundation Trust & Others* [2009] and as yet remain unchallenged. The judgment is long, and the intricacies of eligibility are too long to be discussed in any great detail here. A lengthier, but illuminating, discussion of the complexity of the situation can be found in Fennell (2007).

The main conclusions in the *GJ* case were that the process for determining eligibility for DoLS can be stated as:

- the MHA takes primacy
- there are three questions to consider when determining whether the MHA or DoLS should be used:
  - Is the person within the scope of the MHA?
  - Is the person a mental health patient?
  - Does the person object to being a mental health patient?

## Primacy

As stated above, DoLS was designed to fill a 'gap' in the law for those individuals who were not being detained under the MHA, but did not have the capacity to consent to admission as informal patients, and were therefore detained without the safeguards that would come with formal detention. That the MHA 'takes primacy' means that only these people should be encompassed within the remit of the DoLS; anyone who would, or could, have been detained under the MHA prior to the introduction of the DoLS should still be detained in this way. Anyone who fulfils the criteria for detention under the MHA must be detained under it if detention is considered necessary; DoLS should not be used just because it is perceived to be a less restrictive alternative.

If the situation seems oblique – particularly if the individual appears to lack capacity – then the clinician must ask the three questions posed in Justice Charles's process for determining eligibility for DoLS set out above.

## Is the person within the scope of the MHA?

Schedule 1A states that 'within the scope of the MHA' means that an 'application could be made' and that the person 'could be detained in hospital'. There were several suggestions as to what 'could be detained' meant in real terms; the argument that Justice Charles found most persuasive in *GJ* was the 'decision-maker test' (*GJ v The Foundation Trust & Others*, 2009). It was held that 'could' simply meant that the individual making the decision as regards eligibility should ask themselves 'whether the criteria set by, or the grounds in, ss. 2 or 3 of the MHA are met'; that is, whether the person has a mental disorder which warrants detention. If the person is not within the scope of the MHA, then DoLS must be used to deprive them of their liberty. If the person is within its scope, the clinician must go on to consider whether the person is a mental health patient.

## Is the person a mental health patient?

By far the simplest way to understand whether a person is a 'mental health patient' is to run a 'but for' test. This requires clinicians to ask themselves, 'But for the treatment for a physical disorder unrelated to their mental disorder, does this person need to be in hospital?'. If the answer to that question is 'no' then, despite being within the scope of the MHA, that Act does not need to be used and the person is eligible for DoLS. If it is 'yes', the primacy rule still holds and the clinician must then consider whether the person is an objecting mental health patient.

## Is the person an objecting mental health patient?

If it has been established that a person is within the scope of the MHA and is also a mental health patient, there is one further criterion to establish – is the person objecting? If a person is objecting to receipt of treatment for their mental disorder, or objecting to remaining in hospital to receive the mental health treatment, they will be ineligible for the DoLS, and the MHA must be used.

More recently, in *DN v Northumberland Tyne and Wear NHS Foundation Trust* [2011], DN claimed that, although detained under section 3 of the MHA, he could be discharged from section if arrangements were made under DoLS for him to be accompanied at all times (to stop him buying alcohol). The Upper Tribunal (the higher 'appeal court' of the mental health tribunal service) considered what was meant by being ineligible for DoLS on account of being within the scope of the MHA, in light of the fact that in *GJ* (above) it had been stated that the MHA takes primacy over the MCA.

The judge concluded that DN was eligible for authorisation under the DoLS regime. By taking account of the possibility of a less restrictive option under DoLS it could not be said that MHA detention was necessary. The proposed treatment (i.e. supervision regarding access to alcohol) was not felt to be specialist mental health treatment. However, a letter from the Department of Health to the court that was reproduced during the case stated: 'the Department does not think it would actually be possible to say, in general, which has primacy over the other'.

The outcome of the case clarifies that if DoLS arrangements would be sufficient to meet the patient's needs, the necessity test for detention under the MHA is not met (even if the patient is 'within the scope' of the Act).

# The Deprivation of Liberty authorisation procedure

It is the responsibility of the managing authority to apply for authorisation from the supervisory body for anyone in their care who is or will be deprived of their liberty. The managing authority of a care home or private hospital will be the person registered under Part II of the Care Standards Act 2000. The managing authority for a hospital will be the NHS trust, foundation trust or local health board with authority over the hospital. For care home admissions, the supervisory body will be the local authority where the relevant person ordinarily resides or, if there is no ordinary residence, the local authority of the care home. For hospital admissions, the supervisory body will be the clinical commissioning group (from April 2013) that commissions the care or treatment, or the National Assembly for Wales if the hospital is in Wales or if the care and treatment was commissioned by a Welsh local health board or the National Assembly for Wales.

A managing authority can apply for two kinds of authorisation, standard or urgent. A standard authorisation should be applied for where deprivation of liberty is anticipated. There is a 21-day deadline for concluding the assessment process. The standard authorisation should be the norm. However, if the need is thought to be urgent, a hospital or care home can issue an urgent authorisation, giving their reasons in writing. In this case, a standard authorisation must be obtained before expiry of the urgent authorisation, that is within 7 days.

Once the application has been made, the supervisory body must commission assessments of the person (known as 'the relevant person' in the procedure) and subsequently provide or refuse authorisation for deprivation of liberty.

The managing authority should tell the relevant person's family, friends and carers, a relevant person's representative (see p. 93) and any independent mental capacity advocate (IMCA) already involved, that it has applied for an authorisation of deprivation of liberty, unless impracticable, impossible or undesirable to do so in the interests of the person's health or safety. Anyone involved in the person's care must be consulted about whether or not, in their view, the DoLS is in the person's best interests.

If there is no one suitable to act as the relevant person's representative, the managing authority must inform the supervisory body when it submits its application for a DoLS authorisation. The supervisory body must then instruct an independent mental capacity advocate, under section 39A of the MCA, to represent the person before any assessments can take place.

This information-provision responsibility of the managing authority continues for the time of the authorisation. It includes making provision for any language or communication difficulties that affect the relevant person and/or their representative.

As legislation bestows a statutory duty on hospitals and care homes to be the managing authority for those who may be deprived of their liberty within their institutions, such authorities must ensure that staff: are aware of legislation; contact local DoLS leads if they believe they may be depriving someone of their liberty; ensure that DoLS are considered for every new admission; develop policies and procedures for authorisation requests; maintain contemporaneous records; take all reasonable steps to ensure that the relevant person or their representative understands what authorisation means and how they can apply to the Court of Protection; ensure that any authorisation conditions are met; and monitor individual circumstances.

## Independent mental capacity advocates

An independent mental capacity advocate (IMCA) instructed for the purpose of representing a person for whom a DoLS authorisation is sought has 'additional rights and responsibilities' compared with an IMCA under the MCA process.

They have the right to give information or make submissions to assessors and the assessors must take them into account. They have the right to receive copies of any assessments from the supervisory body, to receive a copy of an urgent and/or a standard authorisation, and to be notified by the supervisory body if it fails to proceed with an authorisation. They have the right to all documentation relating to all assessment processes.

Any differences of opinion between an IMCA and an assessor should be resolved through informal processes, but if there remain areas of conflict, the supervisory body must be informed before any assessment process is finalised. Ultimately, an IMCA can make an application to the Court of Protection for permission to take the relevant person's case to court in connection with a matter relating to the giving or refusal of any authorisation.

Once a relevant person's representative (RPR) is appointed, the duties of an IMCA cease, although this does not prevent an IMCA from taking a case to court, when they must take account of the views of the RPR. Any gaps in the appointment of an RPR require an IMCA.

## *Applying for DoLS*

Figure 5.1 outlines the process of applying for DoLS authorisation. There are six requirements that must be met before a deprivation of liberty can be authorised. Each must be assessed and found positive. The assessments must be carried out by at least two assessors (and two is the usual number), as the best interests requirement and the mental health requirement must be assessed by different individuals. The requirements to be assessed are as follows.

- Age – the person must be 18 or over.
- Mental health – it must be shown that the person suffers from a mental disorder within the meaning of the MHA, including those with an intellectual (learning) disability (without the exclusions contained in the Act). Dependence on drugs or alcohol is not considered to be a disorder or disability of the mind for the purposes of this legislation.
- Mental capacity – it must be shown that the person lacks capacity to consent to the proposed care and treatment.
- Best interests – it must be shown that: (a) a deprivation of liberty is occurring/will occur; and (b) this deprivation of liberty is in the person's best interests.
- Eligibility – this requirement is complicated, but in its simplest terms it must be shown that the person is not currently, is not liable to be nor could be detained under the MHA. The MHA and the DoLS are supposed to refer to different groups, and cannot be applied at will.
- No refusals – it must be shown that the treatment or care proposed as part of the authorisation has not been refused by an existing valid and applicable advance decision made by the person, or by the person's representative under a lasting power of attorney, or by a court appointed deputy.

# Assessors

The best interests and mental health requirements must be assessed by different people, called the best interests assessor and the mental health assessor. The supervisory body has a legal responsibility to select assessors who are both suitable and eligible.

## *The best interests assessor*

The best interests assessor must be a psychologist, nurse or occupational therapist, who has worked for 2 years after professional registration and has undertaken the relevant training to qualify as a best interests assessor. The best interests assessor may also conduct the assessments for age, mental capacity and no refusals. Best interests assessors who have an additional qualification as an approved mental health practitioner under the MHA may also conduct the assessment for eligibility.

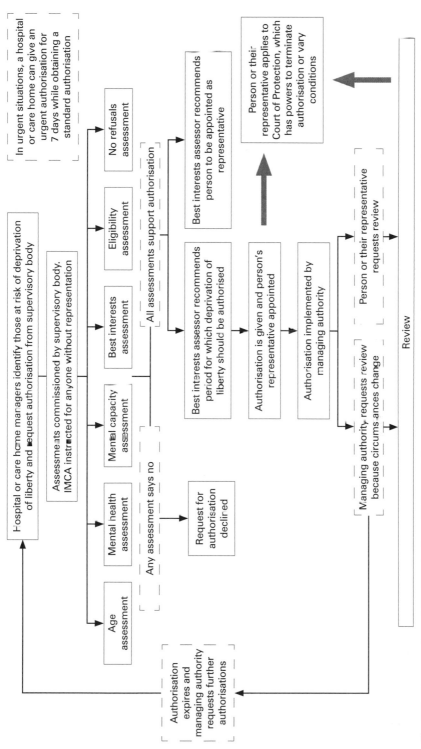

**Fig. 5.1** An overview of the Deprivation of Liberty Safeguards process. IMCA, independent mental capacity advocate (Ministry of Justice, 2008: p. 107. © Crown Copyright 2008).

In conducting the best interests assessment, the assessor must consider and evaluate the care plan, to ensure that the least restrictive option is being pursued in the context of possible harm to the person. The best interests assessor must also seek the views of anyone involved in the person's care, for example family or friends. They must involve the person affected as far as possible and support them in taking part in decision-making, and they must consider the views of the mental health assessor.

The overriding purpose of the best interests assessment is to balance the risk of benefit *v.* the risk of harm, that is whether the deprivation of liberty is a proportionate response to the likelihood of harm occurring.

The best interests assessor has the authority to make recommendations about a proposed deprivation of liberty. Thereafter, a panel of representatives from the local authority sits to make a judgement on the evidence presented by the assessments. It is the supervisory body that has the power to give the authorisation on the basis of receiving the outcome of all the assessments. The best interests assessor must specify how long an authorisation should last and any conditions attached to it, make recommendations for care where a requirement is not met, produce a report outlining their decision and how it was reached, and conduct review assessments at the request of the relevant person, their representative or an IMCA.

## The mental health assessor

Case law of the European Court requires that the mental health assessment be undertaken by a doctor, since 'it must be convincingly shown on the basis of objective medical expertise that the person to be detained is mentally disordered' (*Winterwerp v The Netherlands*, 1979).

The mental health assessor must be approved under section 12 of the MHA or be a registered medical practitioner with 3 years of special experience of mental disorder diagnosis and treatment. In addition, mental health assessors must have completed a mental health assessor training course approved by the Secretary of State. The current relevant course is the Deprivation of Liberty Safeguards Mental Health Assessor Training Programme of the Royal College of Psychiatrists. Refresher training must be undertaken annually.

The mental health assessor is required to assess the impact of a DoLS authorisation on the person's mental health. If possible, the assessor should be someone who knows the person and has experience of their condition. The assessment is not to determine whether the person requires mental health treatment.

It is possible to suspend an authorisation for up to 28 days. This may be necessary if, for example, the person has been detained under the MHA, in a hospital. Supervisory bodies are responsible for this suspension (and its removal) when notified by the managing authority to do so.

## Role of a relevant person's representative

One of the key criticisms put forward by the European Court was that Mr HL had no proper representative who could act as an advocate for him when he was detained at Bournewood Hospital (*HL v The United Kingdom*, 2004). The DoLS process attempts to remedy this by creating the role of a relevant person's representative (RPR).

Once a standard authorisation has been issued, the supervisory body must appoint an RPR as soon as is practicable, to maintain contact and represent the views of the person who has been lawfully deprived of their liberty. The most likely candidate should already have been identified by the best interests assessor, who must consider who is most likely to act in the individual's best interests.

The RPR, who is often a family member, friend or carer of the relevant person, must be able to visit and maintain regular contact with the person, so that they can effectively monitor the authorisation and the continuing fulfilment of its six requirements (age, mental health, mental capacity, best interests, eligibility and no refusals). To be eligible to be appointed as an RPR, an individual must be over 18 and have no financial interest in, nor be the relative of someone with a financial interest in, the relevant person's managing authority. Moreover, they must not be employed by, or provide services to, the care home in which the person resides, or be employed by the hospital in a role that provides care and treatment to the person, or employed to work in the supervisory body in a role that brings them into contact with the relevant person's case.

The RPR may be chosen by the relevant person, if they have capacity to do so, or by a court appointed deputy. The RPR's eligibility is confirmed by the best interests assessor. If the individual put forward is ineligible, an alternative must be chosen by the relevant person, or a court appointed deputy, or the best interests assessor. This RPR is akin to an advocate. The chosen RPR does not need to agree with the DoLS authorisation given.

If the relevant person and best interests assessor cannot choose an appropriate RPR, the supervisory body must make an appointment. This would be a professional position for someone possessing the necessary skills and expertise, not a family member, friend or carer of the relevant person. The individual identified must not be ineligible by virtue of one of the exclusion criteria given above, and must have been issued with an 'appropriate criminal record certificate'. The supervisory body may provide payment for the services provided and may commission such an individual via local advocacy service provider arrangements.

## Review process

Managing authorities monitor the deprivation of liberty, and reviews are carried out by the supervisory body. After the authorisation, the managing authority must ensure compliance with the MCA and the DoLS Code of Practice (Ministry of Justice, 2008) and continuance of the least restrictive regime of care. The same authority provides alternative care where an authorisation is not granted. The supervisory body reviews cases to determine whether a DoLS authorisation is still necessary and removes it if it is not. Further details of the review processes can be found in the Dols Code of Practice (Ministry of Justice, 2008).

## Role of the Court of Protection

Compliance with Article 5(4) of the European Convention on Human Rights, which is the right to speedy access to court to review the lawfulness of any deprivation of liberty, is guaranteed by the expanded remit of the Court of Protection to review authorisations for deprivation of liberty.

The relevant person can make an application, as can someone acting on their behalf, even before a decision is reached about a DoLS authorisation. The Court can make decisions on lawfulness, the person's capacity and what is in the person's best interests.

After an authorisation has been issued, whether standard or urgent, the Court can make decisions relating to qualifying requirements for deprivations of liberty, the period for which an authorisation should be in place, the purpose for which an authorisation is given and the conditions attached to any authorisation. The Court can make an order varying or terminating a standard or urgent authorisation, and can direct the supervisory body to vary or terminate the authorisation.

Some groups have an automatic or unfettered right of access to the Court of Protection: the relevant person, the donor or donee of a lasting power of attorney, a court appointed deputy, a person named in an existing court order to which the application relates, and a person appointed by the supervisory body as the RPR. Any other person may be granted permission by the Court (MCA: section 50).

## How are the safeguards monitored?

The Care Quality Commission (CQC) monitors the manner in which DoLS are operated by hospitals and care homes, seeking to ensure that the safeguards are working properly. It is able to visit hospitals and care homes and talk to patients and residents. Supervisory bodies must disclose information to the CQC as part of the inspection process. The CQC reports annually to the Secretary of State, summarising its activities and findings.

In Wales, the functions of monitoring the DoLS fall to Welsh Ministers, performed on their behalf by the Healthcare Inspectorate Wales and the Care and Social Services Inspectorate Wales.

# References

Department of Health (2005) *'Bournewood' Consultation: The Approach to Be Taken in Response to the Judgement of the European Court of Human Rights in the 'Bournewood' Case*. Department of Health.

Department of Health (2011) *Summary of Two Cases on the Meaning of Deprivation of Liberty: The "MIG and MEG" Case and the "A and C" Case* (Gateway reference: 15723). Department of Health.

Fennell, P. (2007) *Mental Health: The New Law*. Jordans.

Ministry of Justice (2008) *Mental Capacity Act 2005: Deprivation of Liberty Safeguards. Code of Practice to Supplement the Main Mental Capacity Act 2005 Code of Practice*. TSO (The Stationery Office).

Morris, F. & Ruck Keene, A. (2007) *Deprivation of Liberty: The Bournewood Proposals, the Mental Capacity Act 2005 and the Decision in JE v DE and Surrey County Council*. 39 Essex Street.

Scottish Law Commission (2012) *Discussion Paper on Adults with Incapacity (Discussion Paper No. 156)*. TSO (The Stationery Office).

## Cases of the European Court of Human Rights

*DD v Lithuania* [2012] ECHR 254.

*Engel & Others v The Netherlands* (1976) 1 EHRR 647.

*Guzzardi v Italy* (1980) 3 EHRR 333.

*HL v The United Kingdom* [2004] 45508/99 ECHR 471.

*Kedzior v Poland* [2012] ECHR 1809.

*Stanev v Bulgaria* [2012] ECHR 46.

*Storck v Germany* (2005) 43 EHRR 96.

*Winterwerp v The Netherlands* [1979] 6301/73 ECHR 4.

## Domestic cases

*A Primary Care Trust v P & Others* [2009] EW Misc 10 (EWCOP).

*BB v AM* (2010) EWHC 1916 (Fam).

*CC v KK and STCC* [2012] EWHC 2136 (COP).

*Cheshire West and Chester Council v P* [2011] EWCA Civ 1257.

*DN v Northumberland Tyne and Wear NHS Foundation Trust* [2011] 3 UKUT 327 (AAC).

*Dorset CC v EH* [2009] EWHC 784 (Fam)

*G v E (By his litigation friend the Official Solicitor)* [2010] EWHC 621 (COP).

*GJ v The Foundation Trust & Others* [2009] EWHC 2972 (Fam)

*JE v DE and Surrey County Council* [2006] EWHC 3459 (Fam).

*LLBC v TG* [2007] EWHC 2640 (Fam).

*London Borough of Hillingdon v Neary & Another* [2011] EWHC 1377 (COP).

*Surrey County Council v CA & LA & MIG & MEG* [2010] EWHC 785 (Fam).

*P and Q v Surrey County Council* [2011] EWCA Civ 190.

*Re A (Adult); Re C (Child); A Local Authority v A* [2010] EWHC 978 (Fam).

# CHAPTER 6

# Clinical ambiguities in the assessment of capacity

## Rebecca Jacob and Elizabeth Fistein

Legislation pertaining to health, social care and financial decisions on behalf of those without capacity came into being with the introduction of the Mental Capacity Act 2005 (MCA). A Code of Practice, published soon after, appears to give clear and concise guidelines on the management of those without capacity using best interests principles (Department for Constitutional Affairs, 2007). Nonetheless, despite this seemingly explicit guidance there remain dilemmas and uncertainties in the application of the Act in a variety of clinical settings. This may be related to the following observation: although the legal concept of capacity seems unambiguous, and both English and Scottish legislation incorporate similar definitions of it (Mental Capacity Act 2005 and Adults with Incapacity (Scotland) Act 2000), the application of legal tests of capacity in clinical settings is far from straightforward (Herring, 2008). This is evidenced by the statement of Dame Elizabeth Butler-Sloss, in her ruling on the case of Ms B:

> 'The general law on mental capacity is, in my judgment, clear and easily to be understood by lawyers. Its application to individual cases in the context of a general practitioner's surgery, a hospital ward and especially in an intensive care unit is infinitely more difficult to achieve' (Re B (Adult: Refusal of Medical Treatment), 2002).

Medical practitioners have also long voiced their frustrations about the complexity of applying legal tests to clinical situations, as exemplified by the following:

> 'The search for a single test of competency is a search for a Holy Grail. [...] In practice, judgments of competency go beyond semantics or straightforward applications of legal rules; such judgments reflect social considerations and societal biases as much as they reflect matters of law and medicine' (Roth et al, 1977: p. 283).

As described in Chapter 4, the functional test of capacity (Grisso et al, 1997) has now been accepted in many jurisdictions as the most appropriate legal test of capacity. Its use has replaced the status approach, which relies on a person's condition or diagnosis as a marker of competence, and the outcome approach, which focuses on whether or not a patient's decision appears 'sound or reasonable'. The MCA creates a statutory duty to perform a functional assessment of capacity, or the ability to make a particular decision at a particular time, which seems at first to be both clear and precise. However, cases such as *Re C (Adult: Refusal of Medical Treatment)* [1994] show that in some respects capacity lies on a dimensional scale and its determination is not, in clinical practice at least, always a simple black and white issue. As Justice Thorpe comments in his ruling in *Re C*:

> 'If the patient's capacity to decide is unimpaired, autonomy weighs heavier but the further capacity is reduced, the lighter autonomy weighs' *(Re C (Adult: Refusal of Medical Treatment)*, 1994).

The fact that an individual's capacity can be 'reduced' suggests that it is not, in fact, an all or nothing ability. It is the law that imposes a dichotomy (competent *v.* incompetent) on what is arguably a spectrum of ability. There is an expectation that, concerning a specific question and at a specific time, an individual either does or does not have capacity. This decision is based on the balance of probabilities, that it is more likely than not that, at this point in time, this person's ability to make this particular decision is so impaired that they should be judged unable to decide. This lack of certainty, and the requirement to make a binary decision based on an ability usually better understood as moving along a sliding scale, may feel unsatisfactory when treating a patient against their wishes.

How then should clinicians approach cases where the legal test of capacity is difficult to apply? Ideally, legal advice must be easily accessible for cases that appear controversial because of questions relating to the assessment of capacity. The following examples, drawn from case law, typify some of the contentious issues faced by clinicians. The problems considered are: how to respond when the patient seems ambivalent about their own decision; when to intervene in cases of fluctuating capacity; how much weight to give to unusual beliefs; and how to avoid unwittingly adopting a status-based approach to capacity in particular patient groups. They are discussed in some detail, in order to illustrate the current legal position and to provide some guidance for clinicians who encounter similar cases. Finally, the management of self-harm, a situation that often raises all of the issues discussed in this chapter, is reviewed and relevant cases are discussed.

# Ambivalence

Assessing the capacity of people who are ambivalent about treatment can be particularly complex. Ambivalence in this context implies that the individual has difficulties in coming to a decision about the treatment in question and vacillates between accepting or refusing treatment. This may suggest that they are experiencing difficulty with the third component of the capacity test laid down in the MCA: that a person lacks capacity if they unable to use or weigh information relevant to the decision. Alternatively, it may simply indicate that the decision to be made is difficult or finely balanced and that therefore a degree of vacillation might be expected.

A case in point is that of Ms B, a 43-year-old woman who was paralysed from the neck down and sustained only by means of a ventilator (*Re B*, 2002). She refused this intervention shortly after it was introduced, despite being made aware that ventilatory support was necessary to preserve life. The treating team did not accept her refusal of treatment, as they believed they could make a difference to the quality of her life with treatment and that she could not make an informed choice without experiencing the benefits of the proposed rehabilitative procedure. The doctors used the argument that they could not take her decision to discontinue treatment as final because she vacillated in her decision-making process. It is clear that the greater the vacillation in decision-making, the more likely it is that an individual will be regarded as incapable of making that decision. This ambivalence gives rise to several lines of questioning. Is ambivalence *per se* a sign that an individual is incompetent? There is after all an expectation that, if capable, the individual should come to some conclusion regarding treatment. Second, when should a decision be accepted as final? The danger is that health professionals may accept the decision that they consider reasonable, notwithstanding the ambivalence shown. Yet another question arises: should a refusal of life-preserving treatment be automatically suspect? And, given the irreversible consequences of such a decision, how long should a health professional wait for a possible change of heart before the decision is accepted?

In this case, Ms B sought declarations from the High Court stating that she was competent to refuse life-prolonging medical treatment and that the hospital had been treating her unlawfully from the time she had stated her refusal. The judge, Dame Elizabeth Butler-Sloss, identified as the central issue in the case the question of whether Ms B had been competent to refuse ventilation. Starting from the legal presumption that all adults possess capacity, the judge found that Ms B was indeed competent. She consequently granted the declarations sought and made a nominal award of damages against the hospital for trespass to the person, stressing the duty to respect competent patients' refusals of treatment:

> 'I am therefore entirely satisfied that Ms. B is competent to make all relevant decisions about her medical treatment including the decision whether to seek to withdraw from artificial ventilation. Her mental competence is commensurate with the gravity of the decision she may wish to make. [...] I would like to add how impressed I am with her as a person, with the great courage, strength of will and determination she has shown in the last year, with her sense of humour, and her understanding of the dilemma she has posed to the Hospital. She is clearly a splendid person and it is tragic that someone of her ability has been struck down so cruelly. I hope she will forgive me for saying, diffidently, that if she did reconsider her decision, she would have a lot to offer the community at large.' (*Re B (Adult: Refusal of Medical Treatment)*, 2002).

The subsequent withdrawal of ventilation later led to Ms B's death as predicted by the treating clinicians. This ruling serves to illustrate a shift in legal opinion from acceptance of medical paternalism to promotion of personal autonomy. As Dame Butler-Sloss stated:

> 'There is a serious danger, exemplified in this case, of a benevolent paternalism which does not embrace recognition of the personal autonomy of the severely disabled patient.'

It would seem erroneous, on reflection, to assume that some ambivalence when faced with life-preserving healthcare decisions is abnormal or unreasonable in any way. This would imply that difficulty and some degree of vacillation when making hard choices would be synonymous in some way with incapacity. Certainly, a more complex medical intervention would require a greater commitment from the patient when consenting and most usually have more profound health consequences. Accordingly, it would stand to reason that a level of uncertainty, fear and vacillation could be evident and clinicians must take this into account when making assessments of decision-making capacity. In other words, ambivalence should not be assumed equivalent to incapacity. The test is whether or not the patient, as a result of disorder or dysfunction of mind or brain, is unable to weigh the information relevant to the decision (MCA: section 2(1)). The fact that a decision is a difficult one, with life-or-death consequences, that naturally may take some time and careful consideration to make must not, in itself, be taken to mean that the person who is in the unfortunate position of having to make that decision lacks capacity (Gunn, 2009).

## Fluctuating capacity

Another difficulty arises in cases of fluctuating capacity. The ability to make a particular decision at a specific time may be based on a number of factors, such as physical health, intoxication with substances and mental illness, and someone affected by such conditions may be able to make a decision at one time but incapable at another. When an individual is deemed to be incapable, a judgement must be made as to whether treatment can be delayed until the patient is given a chance to recover capacity and review the decision at hand. A case in point is alcohol intoxication, which is a common confounding factor when treatment decisions need to be made for patients who self-harm (Hawton *et al*, 1989). The difficulty is in deciding whether these patients should be treated immediately, in their own best interests, or whether it would be reasonable to wait till they are sober and seek their consent to the necessary treatments. The pivotal deciding factor in these cases would appear to be a clinical rather than a legal decision, and would hinge on whether the situation could be termed an emergency or not.

The case of *Re R (A Minor) (Wardship: Medical Treatment)* [1991] illustrates a medical professional's dilemma when dealing with emergency medical decisions regarding a patient who has fluctuating capacity. The case concerned a 15-year-old girl who had severe mental health problems and who refused the administration of antipsychotic medication. Her capacity was questioned owing to the fact that on occasion she did not appear able to make a fully informed refusal of treatment, although at other times she did appear more lucid and able to make a choice. Lord Donaldson took the opportunity to express his view on the ability of a person with parental responsibility to override an incompetent child's refusal of treatment. He stated that it was clearly in R's best interests to have treatment and, as she was not in a position to give a competent decision because of her fluctuating mental capacity, the decision was taken out of her hands and she was given the necessary treatment. However, under the MCA, fluctuating capacity is by no means considered equivalent to incapacity. The duty to maximise capacity would involve delaying the decision, whenever possible, to allow the patient to decide during a period of lucidity. During such an interval, the patient can make contemporaneous decisions about immediate treatment.

Moreover, the MCA contains provisions that can be used to facilitate the patient's involvement in advance care-planning. First, the issuing of an 'advance decision' could be considered during lucid intervals. Advance decisions allow an individual to refuse a particular treatment, should they become incompetent in the future. What must be highlighted is that advance decisions refer only to the refusal of specific treatments, and cannot compel a clinician to offer a particular type of treatment. It must also be noted that, in the case of a mentally ill patient detained under the Mental Health Act 1983 (MHA), an advance decision to refuse medical treatment for mental disorder may be overridden.

Second, during periods of capacity the patient may nominate another adult as having 'lasting power of attorney', enabling that person to make decisions on behalf of the patient during any further episodes of incapacity. The person nominated will still be required to make decisions in the best interests of the patient but, if they know the patient well, they may be in a better position than the doctor to incorporate the patient's wishes, feelings, beliefs and values into the decision-making process.

Finally, if treatment is needed during a period of incapacity and it is not clinically acceptable to wait for a potential lucid period, best interest principles apply. The treating clinician must make the choice as to the best interests of the patient after ascertaining from relatives, or an independent mental capacity advocate, the previously expressed wishes of the patient (Department for Constitutional Affairs, 2007). This will involve careful consideration of views expressed by the patient during periods of lucidity. Dame Butler-Sloss has described best interests as 'not limited to best medical interests' (Re MB (An Adult: Medical Treatment), 1997), encompassing 'medical, emotional and all other welfare issues' (Re A (Medical Treatment: Male Sterilisation), 2000). Although one would assume that this would be based solely on the patient's declaration related to the treatment decision at hand, so far has the law progressed that there is little that falls outside the jurisdiction of the court, and its determination will be reached by a careful and sympathetic appreciation of all relevant factors.

## Unusual values/belief systems

A further area of complexity is the relevance of values or belief systems that may influence an individual's decision-making capacity. There is an understanding, shaped by case law, that a decision which might be influenced by a set of values or religious beliefs, should be respected. The example of a Jehovah's Witness refusing to accept a blood transfusion on the grounds of religious beliefs is a case in point. Without background knowledge of the dogma on which this belief system is centred, such a stance might make one question the patient's mental state and suspect a mental disorder.

However, what about more idiosyncratic beliefs that may indicate the presence of a mental disorder? Psychiatric delusions, particularly of persecution, might make a patient believe wrongly that a treatment will do him harm rather than good. A patient with psychotic depression might have delusions of guilt or worthlessness (Carpenter *et al*, 2000) and might be convinced that she deserves the illness and is not worthy of help. In some cases, it might be appropriate to use the MHA to provide treatment for the underlying mental disorder. However, not all mentally ill people meet criteria for compulsory treatment under the MHA, which states that the patient must have a mental disorder of a nature and degree that requires hospital treatment, and that this is the least restrictive treatment option. Furthermore, the MHA does not provide any legal justification for the provision of treatment for physical conditions in the absence of consent. If such treatment were required, it would be important to assess whether the delusions affect the patient's decision-making capacity as defined by the MCA. In particular, delusions or cognitive bias arising as a result of serious mental illness may render a patient unable to give appropriate weight to relevant information and so reach a decision.

When a belief system is shared by a group of individuals, it is easier to accept and understand how it might influence decision-making. The problem that confounds clinicians is under what circumstances they should consider an individual's belief system a reason for questioning their capacity to make decisions. This inevitably becomes relevant in the context of a refusal of treatment. As outlined in Chapter 2 of this volume, the MCA imposes a presumption of capacity for all adults. Findings of incapacity can only be made in the context of a disorder or dysfunction of the mind or brain. Generally, it appears to be the case that unless there is an identifiable mental disorder, value systems must, perforce, be accepted.

An example of such a difficulty is to be found in the case of *St George's Healthcare NHS Trust v S* (1993). S, a veterinary nurse and 36 weeks pregnant, was diagnosed with pre-eclampsia severe enough to require hospital admission and induction of labour. She rejected the advice of the doctors because she felt that the pregnancy should proceed without medical intervention. As she refused admission and treatment, she was forcibly admitted to hospital under section 2 of the MHA, a 28-day assessment section. She documented her reasons for refusing to accept treatment in a form, similar to that used in an advance directive:

> 'At the request of Dr Jeffreys, senior registrar, I am writing in an effort to clarify my views, and reason for upholding them so strongly, with regard to medical or surgical intervention in the case of illness. I am a qualified veterinary nurse, and am therefore quite able to comprehend the medical terminology used and feel happy to ask for clarification if an unfamiliar term is used.
>
> I fully understand that pre-eclampsia is a potentially life-threatening condition, i.e. that raised blood pressure may lead to hemorrhage, shock and if untreated death; alternatively death due to total organ failure resulting from inability to compensate.
>
> I have always held very strong views with regard to medical and surgical treatments for myself and particularly wish to allow nature to "take its course" without intervention. I fully understand that, in certain circumstances, this may endanger my life. I see death as a natural and inevitable end point to certain conditions and that natural events should not be interfered with. It is not a belief attached to the fact of my being pregnant, but would apply equally to any condition arising.'

She was transferred from a psychiatric ward to a general hospital and an urgent *ex parte* declaration that it would be lawful to perform a Caesarean section without consent was sought and duly granted. A Caesarean section was performed and S was safely delivered of her baby. Although not specifically relevant to the point in question, it is nonetheless interesting to note that during her period under section 2 of the MHA, she did not receive treatment for any mental disorder.

The Court of Appeal later rejected the defence that S lacked the capacity to consent and concluded:

> 'while pregnancy increases the personal responsibilities of a woman, it does not diminish her entitlement to decide whether or not to undergo medical treatment. Although human, and protected by the law in a number of different ways set out in the judgment in *Re MB*, an unborn child is not a separate person from its mother. Its need for medical assistance does not prevail over her rights. She is entitled not to be forced to submit to an invasion of her body against her will, whether her own life or that of her unborn child depends on it. Her right is not reduced or diminished merely because her decision to exercise it may appear morally repugnant. The declaration in this case involved the removal of the baby from within the body of her mother under physical compulsion. Unless lawfully justified, this constituted an infringement of the mother's autonomy. Of themselves, the perceived needs of the foetus did not provide the necessary justification' (*St George's Healthcare NHS Trust v S, R v Collins, ex parte S*, 1998).

S's value system was clearly pivotal in her decision not to accept treatment for pre-eclampsia, and it would be contentious – and indeed unlawful – to argue that a decision based on a value system is irrational merely because the vast majority of people faced with a similar decision would choose to accept the necessary medical or surgical treatment. It would also appear dubious in this case to have diagnosed a mental disorder when presented with a clear and coherent request that did not appear to either have a delusional basis or be led by a suicidal wish, as might occur in the context of a depressive disorder. However, it is not uncommon for mental illness to underpin an unusual and newly held belief. It would therefore be vital to assess and clearly document the presence or absence of a mental disorder underlying a value system, before either accepting or overriding refusal of treatments. That said, it is important not to jump to the conclusion that the presence of a mental illness that leads to the development of unusual or delusional beliefs will inevitably cause incapacity to make a particular decision. The effect of mental illness on capacity is considered further in the next section.

## Incapacity in vulnerable populations

There is now substantial empirical literature about the capacity of different groups of adults, including those with physical illness, mental illness, dementia and intellectual disabilities, to make decisions, including decisions specifically concerning treatment. Generally, but by no means inevitably, people with mental disorders, particularly psychosis, are more likely than their 'general population' counterparts to experience impairments in their decision-making capacity (Wong et al, 1999, 2000; Bellhouse et al, 2003; Owen et al, 2009). However, there is a danger of applying the status approach to those with mental disorders and erroneously concluding, on the basis of their diagnosis, that they do not have capacity. Just as a number of studies have suggested that patients with mental disorders, particularly psychosis, have difficulty with the consent process, several have highlighted the fact that patients with other mental disorders, such as depression, are well able to participate in the consent process. Research has suggested that conditions affecting insight or understanding of the illness are more likely than others to impair capacity. Psychotic disorders are characterised by their likelihood to distort reality and by a lack of acceptance of illness, and this encroaches on patients' understanding of the existence of their illness and the need for treatment. Conditions such as depression, however, are less likely to distort understanding, although depression and psychosis are not mutually exclusive conditions (Grisso & Appelbaum, 1991, 1995).

A number of replicated studies have suggested that incapacity is more commonly seen among patients with neurological disorders, including dementia and intellectual disabilities (Marson et al, 1996). Studies have also highlighted difficulties with the consent process in those with a variety of medical disorders, usually affecting the higher cognitive functions (Raymont et al, 2004). This is what one would expect, as the functional assessment of capacity requires cognitive abilities to do with reasoning, understanding, memory and executive function.

# Self-harm and treatment consent/refusal

A particularly contentious issue arising not infrequently in emergency medical practice, confounding both physicians and psychiatrists alike, is the treatment of individuals who self-harm. Self-harm has been variously defined and, over the years, the terms deliberate self-harm, intentional self-harm, parasuicide, attempted suicide, non-fatal suicidal behaviour and self- inflicted violence have all been used to describe the act. More recently, the National Institute for Health and Clinical Excellence (NICE) suggested the use of the term 'self-harm', which patients seem to find more acceptable and less pejorative. In guidelines pertaining to the management of self-harm, NICE defines self-harm as 'self-poisoning or injury, irrespective of the apparent purpose of the act' (National Institute for Health and Clinical Excellence, 2004: p. 7). Managing a case of self-harm will sometimes raise all of the issues discussed so far in this chapter: ambivalence, fluctuating capacity, unusual values and the treatment of a vulnerable group prone to be labelled as lacking the capacity to make their own decisions.

Self-harm is a complex behaviour that can best be thought of as a maladaptive response to acute and chronic stress, often but not exclusively linked with thoughts of suicide. Many of those who harm themselves have a severe mental disorder and/or have misused alcohol; it is not uncommon for people who have harmed themselves to refuse treatment, despite attending an emergency department seemingly of their own free will (Hassan *et al*, 1999; Jacob *et al*, 2005). This may seem surprising, but less so when considering the suicidal intent that not uncommonly drives their act of self-harm. However, it must be pointed out that many acts of self-harm are not directly associated with suicidal intent. They are often an attempt to communicate with others, to influence or to secure help as a way of obtaining relief from a difficult and otherwise overwhelming situation or emotional state. The fact that people attend hospital at all may signal their degree of uncertainty or ambivalence about their actions. When viewed in the context of their complex mental processes, this situation seems more easily understood, but in the setting of a busy emergency department, the management of these patients is particularly challenging. It is important to adopt an empathic, non-judgemental approach and to avoid the 'malignant alienation' that can increase risk of subsequent suicide (Mackay & Barrowclough, 2005).

Irrespective of the events leading to an admission to an emergency department, it remains the duty of the treating team to assess the individual's capacity when dealing with refusal of treatment. This process can be pivotal in resolving the conflict that arises between respect for autonomy and the individual's need for care and protection from harm.

People who have recently harmed themselves often have fluctuating capacity owing to the physical effects of their self-harm or the misuse of alcohol. There is sometimes confusion among healthcare professionals regarding the management of patients who refuse treatment, because of the law's disparate treatment of those with mental illness and those with physical illness (Szmukler, 2004). On the face of it, those with physical health needs such as suturing, surgery or the administration of an antidote to self-poisoning must give consent before the procedure is carried out. Refusal by those who have capacity must be respected, although those who lack capacity may still be given emergency treatment if it is judged necessary to their best interests. This was the difficulty faced by the emergency department team involved in a recent well-publicised case involving the death of Kerrie Wooltorton, a young woman who developed renal failure following the deliberate consumption of antifreeze. She had called an ambulance so that she could end her life without discomfort in hospital, rather than alone at home. She refused all active treatment proposed to save her life, and produced a written statement, which made it clear that she wished to refuse treatment even though her death would be the likely consequence. The treating team judged that Ms Wooltorton retained the capacity to make her own decision about treatment and that they could not, therefore, impose treatment to save her life in the absence of her consent.

The reports of this case in the media understandably raised questions and concerns among both physicians and psychiatrists (McLean, 2009; David et al, 2010). Professor Dinesh Bhugra, then Dean of the Royal College of Psychiatrists, sought clarity for practitioners. In response, Professor Louis Appleby, then National Director for Mental Health, sought to clarify the legal duties and powers of doctors in an open letter to the Royal College of Psychiatrists (Appleby, 2009) in which he stated:

> 'on the general issue, there are two key points that I would make. The first is that it has been established (for example by the case of *B v Croydon Health Authority*) that treatment for mental disorder under the Mental Health Act can include treatment of the physical consequences of self-harm which results from that disorder [...] The second point is that it is possible for someone to meet the criteria for detention under the [Mental Health] Act even though they retain the mental capacity to take decisions about their treatment'.

So, as discussed above, competent refusals to accept physical treatment for a mental disorder may sometimes be overridden, using the MHA. The MHA is concerned with a patient's health and safety and also the risk of others, therefore when a section for assessment or treatment is considered, the best interests of more than just the patient are considered. In certain cases brought before the courts, it has been suggested that self-harm is a behavioural extension of an underlying mental illness and should therefore be treated, if the criteria are met, under the aegis of the MHA, even where treatment is refused. The leading case, mentioned by Professor Appleby in his letter on the Wooltorton case, is that of *B v Croydon Health Authority*

[1995], which gave the Court of Appeal the opportunity to review the substantive issues relating to force-feeding under section 63 of the MHA. The case involved the appellant, B, who had a borderline personality disorder coupled with post-traumatic stress disorder. B was admitted under section 3 of the MHA because of her irresistible urge to inflict self-harm. While in hospital she began to refuse food as a method of inflicting self-harm. She was subsequently force-fed using a nasogastric tube, but sought an injunction against this. At the time of the full hearing, Justice Thorpe held that tube-feeding did constitute treatment for B's mental disorder within the meaning of section 63 of the MHA, as it was treatment for the starvation that was a direct sequel of her mental disorder.

This view was further upheld at the Court of Appeal (*B v Croydon Health Authority*, 1995). Lord Justice Hoffmann stated:

> 'It would seem strange to me if a hospital could, without the patient's consent, give him treatment directed to alleviating a psychopathic disorder showing itself in suicidal tendencies, but not without such consent be able to treat the consequences of a suicide attempt.'

He went on to state:

> 'Nursing and care concurrent with the core treatment or as a necessary prerequisite to such treatment or to prevent the patient from causing harm to himself or to alleviate the consequences of the disorder are, in my view, all capable of being ancillary to a treatment calculated to alleviate or prevent a deterioration of the psychopathic disorder.'

This suggests therefore that treatment refusals by competent patients detained under the MHA may not be respected if the treatment relates even quite distantly to a component of their mental disorder. Their Lordships did advise, however, that without the existence of a core treatment, in this case psychoanalytical therapy, tube-feeding would by itself have been unlawful, as would the very detention of the appellant (Keywood, 1995).

Although the consideration of the use of best interests principles was not an issue that was pertinent to the case of B, it would be applicable if the patient concerned lacked capacity. B apparently valued and pursued forms of physical harm, in this case self-starvation, over treatment that could restore her health, perhaps as a means of dealing with difficult emotions in the only way she knew. This unusual evaluation of self-harm could be understood as arising in the context of a mental disorder: borderline personality disorder. Moreover, B's unusual value system could be seen as preventing her from weighing up the information relevant to the decision to accept or refuse treatment for the physical consequences of her self-harm. In other words, a patient detained under the MHA for treatment of a mental disorder could lawfully be given physical treatments using best interests principles if they lacked capacity to consent to such treatment. Furthermore, if a patient in an emergency department is found to lack capacity and to need treatment in their best interests for the consequences of self-harm, then this treatment could be given under the provisions of the MCA even if the MHA did not apply. Nonetheless, it is important to remember the presumption of capacity for all adults, including those who self harm. Research evidence shows that a significant proportion of people who present to the emergency department following self-harm do retain the capacity to make decisions about medical treatment and, furthermore, that relatively simple interventions can be used to improve impaired decision-making capacity in those who initially fail the test laid out in the MCA (Jacob *et al*, 2005).

# Conclusion

Despite legal guidance in the form of the Mental Capacity Act 2005 and the Mental Health Act 1983, as amended in 2007, there remains some ambiguity in the management of individuals who either lack capacity and/or have a mental disorder, particularly when they refuse treatment. It is therefore important that psychiatrists are confident of the general principles guiding the management of patients who need treatment under either mental health or mental capacity legislation, but remain prepared to take advantage of the legal support systems available in difficult or controversial cases.

# References

Appleby, L. (2009) Letter to Royal College of Psychiatrists: Mental Health Act 1983 and the treatment of the physical consequences of self-harm. Royal College of Psychiatrists.

Bellhouse, J., Holland, A. J., Clare, I. C. H., *et al* (2003) Capacity-based mental health legislation and its impact on clinical practice: 2) treatment in hospital. *Journal of Mental Health Law*, **9**, 24–37.

Carpenter, W. T., Jr, Gold, J. M., Lahti, A. C., *et al* (2000) Decisional capacity for informed consent in schizophrenia research. *Archives of General Psychiatry*, **57**, 533–538.

David, A., Hotopf, M., Moran, P., *et al* (2010) Mentally disordered or lacking capacity? Lessons for management of serious deliberate self-harm. *BMJ*, **7**, 341.

Department for Constitutional Affairs (2007) *Mental Capacity Act 2005: Code of Practice*. TSO (The Stationery Office).

Grisso, T. & Appelbaum, P. S. (1991) Mentally ill and non-mentally ill patients' abilities to understand informed consent disclosures for medication: preliminary data. *Law and Human Behaviour*, **15**, 377–388.

Grisso, T. & Appelbaum, P. S. (1995) The MacArthur Treatment Competence Study. III: Abilities of patients to consent to psychiatric and medical treatments. *Law and Human Behaviour*, **19**, 149–174.

Grisso, T., Appelbaum, P. S. & Hill-Fotouhi, C. (1997) The MacCAT-T: a clinical tool to assess patients' capacities to make treatment decisions. *Psychiatric Services*, **48**, 1415–1419.

Gunn, M. (2009) Hospital treatment for incapacitated adults: Re P. *Medical Law Review*, **17**, 274–281.

Hassan, T. B., MacNamara, A. F., Davy, A., *et al* (1999) Lesson of the week: managing patients with deliberate self-harm who refuse treatment in the accident and emergency department. *BMJ*, **319**, 107–109.

Hawton, K., Fagg, J. & McKeown, S. P. (1989) Alcoholism, alcohol and attempted suicide. *Alcohol and Alcoholism*, **24**, 3–9.

Herring, J. (2008) Entering the fog: on the borderlines of mental capacity. *Indiana Law Journal*, **83** (4), article 16.

Jacob, R., Clare, I. C., Holland, A., *et al* (2005) Self-harm, capacity, and refusal of treatment: implications for emergency medical practice. A prospective observational study. *Emergency Medical Journal*, **22**, 799–802.

Keywood, K. (1995) *B v Croydon Health Authority* 1994, CA: force-feeding the hunger striker under the Mental Health Act 1983. *Web Journal of Current Legal Issues*, (3).

Mackay, N. & Barrowclough, C. (2005) Accident and emergency staff's perceptions of deliberate self-harm: attributions, emotions and willingness to help. *British Journal of Clinical Psychology*, **44**, 255–267.

Marson, D. C., Chatterjee, A., Ingram, K., *et al* (1996) Toward a neurological model of competency: cognitive predictors of capacity to consent in Alzheimer's disease using three different legal standards. *Neurology*, **46**, 666–672.

McLean, S. (2009) Advance directives and the case of Kerrie Wooltorton. *BMJ Blogs*, 1 October.

National Institute for Health and Clinical Excellence (2004) *Self-Harm: The Short-Term Physical and Psychological Management and Secondary Prevention of Self-Harm in Primary and Secondary Care (NICE Clinical Guideline CG16)*. NICE.

Owen, G. S., David, A. S., Richardson, G., *et al* (2009) Mental capacity, diagnosis and insight. *Psychological Medicine*, **39**, 1389–1398.

Raymont, V., Bingley, W., Buchanan, A., *et al* (2004) Prevalence of mental incapacity in medical inpatients and associated risk factors: cross-sectional study. *Lancet*, **364**, 1421–1427.

Roth, L. H., Meisel, A. & Lidz, C. W. (1977) Tests of competency to consent to treatment. *American Journal of Psychiatry*, **134**, 279–284.

Szmukler, G. (2004) Mental health legislation is discriminating and stigmatising. In *Every Family in the Land: Understanding Prejudice and Discrimination against People with Mental Illness* (rev. edn) (ed. A. Crisp), pp. 287–290. Royal Society of Medicine Press.

Wong, J. G., Clare, I. C. H., Gunn, M. J., *et al* (1999) Capacity to make health care decisions: its importance in clinical practice. *Psychological Medicine*, **29**, 437–446.

Wong, J. G., Clare, I. C. H., Holland, A. J., *et al* (2000) The capacity of people with a 'mental disability' to make a health care decision. *Psychological Medicine*, **30**, 295–306.

## Case law

*B v Croydon Health Authority* [1995] 1 All ER 683.

*Re A (Medical Treatment: Male Sterilisation)* [2000] 1 FLR 549, [2000] 1 FCR 193.

*Re B (Adult: Refusal of Medical Treatment)* [2002] 2 All ER 449.

*Re C (Adult: Refusal of Medical Treatment)* [1994] 1 All ER 819.

*Re MB (An Adult: Medical Treatment)* [1997] 2 FCR 541.

*Re R (A Minor) (Wardship: Medical Treatment)* [1991] 4 All ER 177 CA.

*St George's Healthcare NHS Trust v S* [1993] 3 All ER 673.

*St George's Healthcare NHS Trust v S, R v Collins, ex parte S* (1998) 44 BMLR 160 (CA).

# Index

Compiled by Linda English

Adults with Incapacity (Scotland) Act 2000 6–7, 96
advance decisions to refuse treatment 9, 54, 60–61, 69–71
  applicability 69, 70
  best interests 35, 40, 43, 44
  healthcare records 71
  life-sustaining treatment 40, 45, 59, 69, 70
  mental disorders 71, 100
  validity 69, 70
  witnesses 70
advance statements 45–46
alcohol misuse 99, 104, 105
anorexia nervosa 28
artificial nutrition and hydration 59, 71, 75
assessment of capacity 15–32
  clinical ambiguities 96–108
    ambivalence about treatment 97–99, 104
    fluctuating capacity 99–101, 104, 105
    self-harm 104–107
    unusual values/belief systems 101–103, 104, 106
    vulnerable populations 103–104
  cognitive tests 27
  Court of Protection 55
  definition of mental incapacity 20–25
    ability to make decision 21–25
    appreciation 25–26
    diagnostic threshold 20–21
    expressing choice 24–25
    reasoning 26
    retaining information 23, 25
    understanding 21–23, 27
    weighing or using information 23–24, 26, 97
  difficult-to-assess groups 28
  enhancement of capacity 29–30
  functional approach 16–17, 96–97, 103–104
  information necessary for 17–20
    choice put in straightforward way 17

    communication barriers 19
    concern that patient coerced 19–20
    exact nature of decision 17
    history of refusal 18–19
    number of options 17–18
    risks/benefits with each option 18
    urgency of decision 18
  outcome approach 96
  pertain to specific decision 16–17
  reliability of assessments 27
  research on 25–28
  risk-relativity concept 29
  status approach 96, 97, 103
  thresholds for capacity 28–29
  when to assess 15–16
  who is responsible 16
  written information 30
assisted suicide 40, 43–44, 69
attorney *see* enduring powers of attorney; lasting powers of attorney
autonomy principle 3, 4
  anorexia nervosa 28
  life-sustaining treatment 43, 99
  limitations to 5
  relational 50
  *v.* beneficence 4

*B v Croydon Health Authority* 105–106
*BB v AM* 81
belief systems, unusual 101–103
beneficence principle 3, 4
best interests 17, 33–53, 96
  acts in connection with care or treatment 57, 59, 60
  assessment 59
  assessor 90–92, 93
  checklist 35–51
    all relevant circumstances 36–37, 41
    avoiding discrimination 36
    consulting others 47–50
    encourage participation 38–40, 57
    life-sustaining treatment 40–44
    making judgement 51

person's views  40, 44–47, 57, 100
   regaining capacity  38
   restricting rights and acting reasonably
     50–51
  Court of Protection  10, 44, 51, 55
  decision maker  48, 50, 51, 57, 59, 60
  deprivation of liberty  90–92
  deputies  69
  meaning  33–35
  necessity doctrine  5, 6
  not defined in MCA  33, 34
  proxy decision-making  34, 48
  self-harm  105, 106–107
  substituted judgement  34, 35, 48
bioethical approach  2, 3, 6
borderline personality disorder  106
Bournewood gap  78, 84, 86, 93

Caesarean section  102
capacity
  defined  2, 20–27
  fluctuation  30, 99–101, 104, 105
  presumption of  15
  regaining  38
capacity assessment *see* assessment of
  capacity
care, duty of  58
care homes: deprivation of liberty  78, 82,
  88, 93
Care Quality Commission  94
care or treatment, acts in connection with
  50, 54, 55–61
carers
  acts in connection with care or treatment
   56, 57
  consultee  73
  paid  51, 56
  patient coerced  19–20
case law  1, 5, 11, 77
  Deprivation of Liberty Safeguards  80, 81,
   92
  difficult-to-assess groups  28
  European  80, 92
  US  25
*CC v KK and STCC*  55, 83–84
*Cheshire West and Chester Council v P*  83–84
Children Act 1989:  66
children and adolescents  66, 80, 100
clinical trials  72
Code of Practice  54, 55
  acts in connection with care or treatment
   55–57, 60
  best interests  33, 96
  best interests checklist  35–51
  lasting powers of attorney  61, 63

cognitive impairment  27, 103–104
cognitive tests  27
coma  24
common law  43, 58, 69
communication barriers  19, 24–25
confidentiality  48
consent  15
  advance decisions and  69
  doctrine of necessity and  5–7
  informed  60, 72, 73
court appointed deputies  66, 67–69
  acts in connection with care or treatment
   56, 57
  best interests  51, 69
  neglect  75
  Office of the Public Guardian  10, 68
  property and affairs  69
  research consultee  74
Court of Protection  54, 66–69
  acts in connection with care or treatment
   57, 59–60
  advance decisions  69
  appointees  67
  best interests  10, 44, 51, 55
  deprivation of liberty  80, 89, 94
  visitors  55, 68
  wills  62

deafness  19
decision maker  48, 50, 51, 57, 59, 60, 75
decision-maker test  87
decision-making
  ability to make decision  21–25
  gravity of consequences  29
  information for  17–20
  proxy  34, 48
  support in  29–30
  types of  51
decisions
  excluded  54, 71–72
  life-changing  57
  unwise  15, 16, 28
definitions of mental incapacity  21–27
delirium  30, 58
delusions  23, 26, 101, 103
dementia  79, 103
  assessment of capacity  15, 16, 23, 27
  best interests  39, 42–43, 50
deontological theories  3
depression  23, 24, 101, 103
Deprivation of Liberty Safeguards (DoLS)
  78–95
  application for  90
  authorisation procedure  88–90
  best interests assessor  90–92, 93

cases 95
Court of Protection 80, 94
eligibility for 8
    is person an objecting mental health
        patient 87–88
    is person mental health patient 87
    is person within scope of MHA 87
    primacy 86–87
happiness 81–82
independent mental capacity advocate 89
managing authority 88–89, 93–94
or Mental Health Act 86–88
mental health assessor 92
monitoring of safeguards 94
normality approach 82–83, 84
relevant person's representative (RPR)
    89, 93
restraint 58–59
review process 93–94
Scotland 84
standard authorisation 88, 94
supervisory body 88, 89, 92, 93, 94
urgent authorisation 88, 94
Wales 88, 94
what constitutes 80–86
    context/setting 82–85
    family contact 85
    mental health setting 84–85
    objection 81–82
who may be subject to 79–80
deputies see court appointed deputies
diabetes 18
diagnostic threshold 20–21
DN v Northumberland Tyne & Wear NHS
    Foundation Trust 87–88
donation of organ/bone marrow 59
do not attempt resuscitation order 59

electroconvulsive therapy (ECT) 71, 75
emergencies 60, 75
    best interests 44
    fluctuating capacity 99–100
    research 74
    self-harm 104–107
emotions, strong 20–21, 28
enduring powers of attorney 51, 61, 66
Enduring Powers of Attorney Act 1985: 61
equal consideration principle 21, 27, 36
ethics, medical 2–4, 42, 43
European Convention on Human Rights
    (ECHR)
    Article 5: 78–79, 83, 84, 94
    Article 8: 85
    Human Rights Act 1998: 78
European Court of Human Rights 58

Deprivation of Liberty Safeguards 78, 82,
    83, 92, 93
euthanasia 40, 41, 69
excluded decisions 54, 71–72

families 30, 56
    best interests 33–34, 48–50, 59
    contact and Deprivation of Liberty
        Safeguards 85
    deputies 68
    patient coerced 19–20
    relationship decisions 71
    research 73

G v E 85
General Medical Council guidance 45
GJ v The Foundation Trust 82, 86, 87
GJ v The Foundation Trust and Others 11–13

Hippocratic Oath 3
HL v The United Kingdom 78–79, 85, 93
hospitals
    deprivation of liberty 78, 82, 88
    general hospital 17
human rights 43
Human Rights Act 1998: 2, 78, 85
Human Tissue Act 2004: 74

ill-treatment or neglect offence 54, 75–76
impulse control, disturbance of 23–24
independent mental capacity advocate
    (IMCA) 9–10, 11, 48, 54, 56, 74–75, 89
independent mental health advocate 11
information
    appreciation 25–26
    reasoning 26
    retaining 23, 25
    understanding 21–23, 27
    weighing or using 23–24, 26, 97
    written 30
intellectual disability
    assessment of capacity 15, 16, 103
    best interests 38, 39
    Deprivation of Liberty Safeguards 79, 90
interpreters 19, 30

JE v DE and Surrey County Council 80, 81, 82
Jehovah's Witness 101
justice principle 3

language difficulties 19
lasting powers of attorney (LPAs) 9, 54,
    61–65
    acts in connection with care or treatment
        56, 57

best interests 35, 40, 41, 48, 51, 100
Court of Protection 66
fiduciary duty 62
general rules governing 61–62
how to create 64–65
neglect 75
Office of the Public Guardian 10
paid 62
personal welfare (health and welfare)
    attorney 61, 63–64, 71
property and affairs attorney 61, 62–63,
    64
research consultee 74
restrictions on 63
will 62
Law Commission 1, 7–8, 10
law reports 14
least restrictive option 11, 18, 79
liberty, deprivation of
restraint 58
*see also* Deprivation of Liberty Safeguards
    (DoLS)
life-sustaining treatment
advance refusal of treatment 40, 45, 59,
    69, 70
ambivalence about 98–99
best interests checklist 40–44
lasting powers of attorney 40, 63
*LLBC v TG* 82, 85
locked-in syndrome 25
*London Borough of Hillingdon v Steven Neary &
    Another* 85

MacArthur Competence Assessment Tool
    for Treatment (MacCAT-T) 26–27, 28
McArthur Foundation definition of mental
    capacity 25–27
*Making Decisions* report 8
managing authority 88–89, 93–94
mania 23
*Marshall v Curry* 6, 60
medical ethics 2–4, 42, 43
medical treatment
for mental disorder 71, 100
serious 75
mental capacity: definitions 20–27
Mental Capacity Act 2005 (MCA)
Code of Practice *see* Code of Practice
development 7–8
and Mental Health Act 10–13, 17
Part 1: 54
Part 2: 54–55
preliminary provisions 55–61
principles 15, 16, 28, 33
schedule 1A 86, 87

sections
    section 1: 8
    section 4: 33
    section 4(1): 36
    section 4(2): 36–37
    section 4(3): 38
    section 4(4): 39
    section 4(5): 40, 41
    section 4(6): 45, 46, 47, 59
    section 4(7): 47
    section 4(9): 50
    section 4(11): 37
    section 5: 50, 54, 55, 56, 59
    section 6: 50–51, 54, 55, 58
    sections 7 and 8: 54, 55
    sections 9 to 14: 54, 61
    sections 15 to 23: 54, 66
    sections 24 to 26: 54
    sections 27 to 29: 54
    sections 30 to 34: 54, 72–73
    sections 35 to 41: 54
    sections 42 to 43: 54, 55
    section 44: 54, 75
    sections 45 to 56: 54
    sections 57 to 60: 55
    section 61: 55
    section 62: 40
    section 64(5): 83
summary of provisions 9–10
mental capacity assessment *see* assessment
    of capacity
mental disorder
definition 11
Deprivation of Liberty Safeguards 79, 90
medical treatment for 71, 100
severe 15, 17, 104
status approach and 103
Mental Health Act 1983 (MHA)
2007 amendments 6–7, 78, 79
Deprivation of Liberty Safeguards and
    78–88
and Mental Capacity Act 10–13, 17
Part 4: 64, 71, 75
sections:
    section 2: 87, 102
    section 3: 87
    section 58A: 64, 71
    section 63: 105–106
    section 131: 78
status approach 17
unusual values/beliefs 101, 102, 103
mental health assessor 92
*Mentally Incapacitated Adults and Decision-
    Making: An Overview* consultation paper
    7–8

mind or brain, disorder of 11, 20–21
Mini-Mental State Examination (MMSE) 27
*Murray v McMurchy* 6

necessity doctrine 56, 78
  consent and 5–7
neglect 54, 75–76
negligence 60
neurological disorders 103
non-maleficence principle 3

Office of the Public Guardian 65
  deputies 10, 68
  lasting powers of attorney 10, 61–62, 63,
    64, 65
overdose 24, 28

*P and Q v Surrey County Council* 81, 82, 83, 84
pain, severe 30
paternalism, medical 4, 13, 99
personality disorders 28, 106
person's age, appearance, condition or
  behaviour 21, 36
Preferred Priorities for Care document 45
presumption of capacity 15
*A Primary Care Trust v P* 85
principlism 3
protection imperative 55
proxy decision-making 34, 48
psychotic disorders 24, 99–100, 101, 103
Public Guardian 10, 55, 67

*R v Newington* 76
*R (Burke) v General Medical Council* 45
*Re A (Medical Treatment: Male Sterilisation)*
  100
*Re A and Re C* 82–83
*Re B (Adult: Refusal of Medical Treatment)* 96,
  98–99
*Re C (Adult: Refusal of Medical Treatment)* 24,
  97
*Re F (Mental Patient: Sterilisation)* 7
*Re K, Re F* 63
*Re MB (An Adult: Medical Treatment)* 100

*Re R* 99–100
*Re T (Adult)* 5
*Re Y (Mental Incapacity: Bone Marrow
  Transplant)* 59
regaining capacity 38
religious beliefs 101
research 54, 56, 72–74
  on assessment of mental capacity 25–28
  consultee 73, 74
  research ethics committees 73
  therapeutic or non-therapeutic
    intervention 72–73
restraint 58–59

*St George's Healthcare NHS Trust v S* 101–102
sedation 58
self-harm 20–21, 99, 104–107
State benefits 67
status approach 17, 96, 97, 103
sterilisation 7, 60, 100
*Storck v Germany* 80, 85
suicide 104
  assisted 40, 43–44, 69
supervisory body 88, 89, 92, 93, 94
surgery 6, 59

testamentary capacity 15
third party 15, 59

unconsciousness 5
urgent treatment *see* emergencies
US definition of mental capacity 25–27
utilitarianism 3

value-based practice 49
values 4, 44–47
  statements 45
  unusual 101–103, 104, 106
voting rights 72
vulnerable populations 15–16, 103–104

*Who Decides?* Green Paper 8
*Winterwerp v The Netherlands* 92